HELP YOUR
CHILD OR TEEN
GET BACK ON TRACK

"Back on Track will save families time and money in the short run, and possibly even lives in the long one. Written by a gifted therapist in a jargon-free, reader-friendly, non-judgmental style, it is easy to envision this work as an invaluable tool, treasured by parents, teachers, and coaches who aspire to instill mental as well as physical health in the children they care for and about."

—*Madeleine Blais, Pulitzer Prize winning author of* In These Girls, Hope is a Muscle

"Written by a master clinician, this book performs magic: it is both encyclopedic and brief. It is also authoritative, rich, interesting, and immensely informative and useful to all who care about the mental health of children."

—*Edward Hallowell MD, author of* The Childhood Roots of Adult Happiness

"Dr. Talan provides parents with an extremely useful model to organize their thinking about the issues (both normal and problematic) that underlie child development. His book is like a navigational system to help parents through the sometimes difficult journey of child-rearing… For parents who want a useful way to evaluate whether their child is developmentally on track, this is an excellent resource. It also is rich in suggestions for what do if a child is not on track."

—*Barbara Miller PhD, Licensed School Psychologist and Educational Psychologist*

"This well-written, accessible advice book is perfect for parents with teen worries, who don't have ready access to a friendly neighborhood child and adolescent psychiatrist. This book will top their list because of this author's uniquely comforting blend of authority, common sense, warmth and wisdom."

—*Kyle Pruett MD, Clinical Professor of Child Psychiatry and Director of Medical Studies at the Yale University Child Study Center, Yale University School of Medicine*

"There are many books for the consumer out there about psychiatric topics. But they are not all created equal. Dr. Talan has written a book that truly speaks the language of parents without over-simplifying concepts. As a reader, you sense the intelligence, warmth and expertise emanating from each page. Reading this book is like having an excellent child psychiatrist available to answer all of your most pressing questions 24 hours a day. And not only is it eminently readable, but it is encyclopedic in scope. I can't imagine any question that a parent may have about their children that this book would not answer. I can't wait to start recommending it to parents in my practice. It will provide great solace to many."

—*Daniel Carlat MD, Assistant Clinical Professor of Psychiatry at Tufts University School of Medicine, Boston, MA*

HELP YOUR CHILD OR TEEN GET BACK ON TRACK

What Parents and Professionals Can Do for Childhood Emotional and Behavioral Problems

Kenneth H. Talan MD

Jessica Kingsley Publishers
London and Philadelphia

First published in 2008
by Jessica Kingsley Publishers
116 Pentonville Road
London N1 9JB, UK
and
400 Market Street, Suite 400
Philadelphia, PA 19106, USA

www.jkp.com

Disclaimer: The information in this book is for educational purposes and does not constitute medical advice; nor is it a substitute for discussion between patients and their doctors. Always consult your doctor before taking any of the medication described in this book.

Library of Congress Cataloging in Publication Data
A CIP catalog record for this book is available from the Library of Congress

British Library Cataloguing in Publication Data
A CIP catalogue record for this book is available from the British Library

ISBN 978 1 84310 870 2

Printed and bound in the United States by
Thomson-Shore, Inc.

*To past, present, and future parents committed
to the path of helping their children's lives be safe,
healthy, joyful, and peaceful.*

*The value of marriage is not that adults produce
children but that children produce adults.*

Peter de Vries, American novelist (1910–1993)

ACKNOWLEDGMENTS

For me, the truth of the expression that it takes a whole village to raise a child also applies to writing this book. Although I did the writing, a whole village of people guided, supported, and encouraged me along the way. This includes my colleagues who read early drafts and offered content suggestions about the book, editors who helped to shape the clarity and focus of the book, and the family and friends who tolerated my preoccupation with the book and were encouraging about the work and my steps to publish it. It also includes the parents and children who came to me for help and taught me as I helped them, my teachers and colleagues in psychiatry, child psychiatry, psychoanalysis, Buddhist psychology, and somatic experiencing therapy. And most appreciatively, this includes my two daughters, Deb and Susa, and my wife, Kitty, who have shared with me in the joys and the painful hard work of being a parent and growing up. All these people share in the good of this book and I alone am responsible for any errors or misguidance. Below I list some particular people who helped in specific ways.

Heather Hornik, PhD was an extremely helpful resource for valuable information and wise suggestions regarding Chapter 6 on psychological testing. Jay Indik, MSW, Meg Seiler, MSW, Dennis Rosen, MD, Peter Kenny, MD, Jonathan Schwab, MD, Deb King, MSW, Tom Plaut, MD, Ella Kusnetz, Jon Crispin, Cynthia Monahon, PhD, Edward Plimpton, PhD, and Madeline Blais, PhD, all made many useful, practical suggestions regarding various aspects of the book. Steven Dashef, MD, John Hornik, PhD, Daniel Charlat, MD, Robert Alberti, PhD, Catherine Rule, MEd, the staff at the Cutchins residential program and Children's Clinic, the Wednesday reading group, members of the Havurah, and men's group all provided support and were good sounding boards regarding various issues. Suzanne Plaut was wonderfully skilled in shaping my sentences and paragraphs so they more clearly expressed my ideas. She helped turn a crammed manuscript into an accessible book. My wife Kitty encouraged me during the murky times, listened to my endless chatter during the creative times, and nurtured me throughout.

> I expect to pass through the world but once. Any good therefore that I can do, or any kindness I can show to any creature, let me do it now. Let me not defer it, for I shall not pass this way again.
>
> Stephen Grellet, French/American religious leader (1773–1855)

CONTENTS

List of Tables

INTRODUCTION

Is this book for you?

I wrote this book mainly for parents who want to consult with an expert in child mental health treatment but haven't yet made the phone call or had an appointment.

- You may be worried about your preschooler who is having temper tantrums or who, despite having once been toilet trained, has recently started soiling her underclothes.

- Or perhaps your child is a third to fifth grader who seems impulsive and hyperactive, anxious, or depressed, and his teacher recently said that he wasn't learning at the pace she would expect.

- Maybe your child is an adolescent who is overly preoccupied with food and body weight, engaging in self-abusive behavior, or having troublesome mood swings and erratic behavior.

All parents worry and suffer when their son or daughter is in distress. You try everything you can think of to help. Generally, parents only consider a child mental health consultation when the usual ways of helping the child aren't working anymore. A parent who decides to seek professional support may worry about where to turn for help, and thus feel at the mercy of circumstances. So, specifically, how will this book be helpful? This book is for you if:

- you are concerned about your child's emotions and behavior, and want help figuring out what you can do to help (Chapters 1–5)

- you are thinking about getting professional help for you and your child, but do not know where to begin (Chapter 7)

- someone has suggested that your child should have a "psychological evaluation" but you do not know what that involves (Chapter 6)

- you are wondering how to evaluate particular treatment recommendations someone made for your child (Chapters 8–11)

- your child is already receiving treatment and you do not know how to judge it (Chapters 8–11)
- you have concerns about the costs of mental health care, questions about the practical matters of treatment, or want a book/internet resource list (Chapter 12 and the Appendix).

This book is also for pediatricians who want to consult with a child psychiatrist about a preschooler, school-aged child, or adolescent but have not been able to. Pediatricians can give this book as a resource to parents who have questions about emotional and behavioral difficulties of their child or adolescent.

In addition, this book is a resource for non-medical professionals, such as clinical social workers, psychologists, and counselors, in the field of child mental health treatment. It deals with issues like medical treatment, psychological testing, and perspectives for understanding and treating particular symptoms (such as anxiety, bullying, mood swings, and tantrums).

I would welcome your comments and suggestions about the book at: www.backontrack.kentalan.com.

How to use this book

Below, I describe the contents of each chapter, so you can quickly look up specific information. For each chapter, I recommend that you first read the introduction and organization, which give specific ideas to keep in mind as you read the remaining information.

You can also read through the book from beginning to end. The chapters follow the stages you might go through as you try to figure out how to help your child get back on track. First, you discover something is not right. Then you try to make sense of your child's difficulty and figure out what you can do yourself. If you decide to seek professional help, the second section of the book takes you through the stages of looking for, understanding, and judging treatment.

What's in this book?

The book is divided into two sections. **Section I** (Chapters 1–5) addresses things you can do on your own to understand and help your child.

Chapter 1, *What to Do When You Think Your Child Has a Problem*, takes you through questions and answers to help you think more clearly and carefully about your child's emotional state or behavior. The answers and examples may also help you begin to determine whether to seek professional help.

Chapter 2, *The Red Flags: An Alphabetical List of Symptoms*, lists specific symptoms you may be concerned about: emotions (anxiety, depression, hostility, and shame) or behaviors (bullying, drug use, fighting, and impulsivity) that caught your attention. I discuss each symptom from several points of view, generally including a psychological perspective. I offer some practical ways to respond to your child on a personal level and, sometimes, on the topic of whether professional treatment makes sense, including what kind might be appropriate.

Chapter 3, *Disruptions in Development: The Whole Child*, helps you see your child's problem through a framework that takes into account your child's age and the many tasks that are part of growing up at that particular age. This chapter balances out the "red flag" symptom approach from Chapter 2.

I discuss four age groups: toddler, preschooler, school-aged child, and adolescent. Your child's symptoms have roots in a delay, disruption, or distortion of a normal stage or task in growing up. Therefore, for each age, I discuss four broad categories of developmental tasks involved in growing up: managing the body, modulating emotions, engaging in relationships, and acquiring knowledge about the world (processing information). The developmental perspective helps you think more clearly about which growing up task is likely to be a part of your child's difficulties and how you might best address those difficulties.

Chapter 4, *Ten Steps to Help Your Child Get Back on Track*, covers important ideas and actions to keep in mind no matter what problem your child is having. These suggestions will help you and your child become more connected to one another and more resilient for the task of getting back on track, regardless of whether a professional is involved.

Chapter 5, *Coping With Your Feelings When Your Child Suffers*, discusses the kinds of emotional experiences you may have—guilt, shame, fear, anger, and sadness—when your child has psychological and behavioral difficulties. I suggest a "Parent's Serenity Prayer" to help you cope with the pain caused by not being able to fulfill all your hopes to protect and care for your child.

Section II (Chapters 6–12) addresses what you need to know to make good use of professional resources that can help your child. But I first provide a very brief overview of the changes in child mental health treatment since 1975 to help you better understand how the child mental health system works today. I also critique the current prominence given to the biological/pharmacological perspective in the treatment of children's difficulties.

Chapter 6, *Evaluation and Testing: Why, What, Who, and Where?* discusses what is involved in an evaluation with different kinds of specialists. I emphasize psychological and neuropsychological evaluation and testing, since that is most confusing for parents. I clarify what these tests are and why they are used.

Chapter 7, *Questions about Treatment: Who Are the Helpers and Where Are They?* addresses the complex task of finding the correct mental health specialist to treat your child. You will learn about different types of clinicians, what type of training and expertise each has, and what distinguishes one type of clinician from another. This information will help you find the kind of clinician who best fits your child's needs, and help you have realistic expectations of what a particular clinician can provide. I also describe different types of places where your child can get treatment.

Chapter 8, *Psychotherapy and Its Side Effects*, offers an overview of each type of individual therapy (cognitive behavioral, dialectical behavioral, psychodynamic, interpersonal, and psychoanalytic) as well as the non-individual psychotherapies (group, family, dialectical behavior therapy skills group). This is followed by a FAQ (frequently asked questions) section that addresses common concerns parents come across when a child is in psychotherapy. The chapter ends with a discussion of side effects that can come up in the course of psychological treatment.

Chapter 9, *Medications and Their Side Effects*, informs you about the range of available pharmacological treatments. I discuss the guiding principles involved in the medical treatment of children and answer common questions that may come up. I use psychological terms to explain how medication can help with behavioral and emotional problems.

Chapter 10, *Complementary and Alternative Therapies and Their Side Effects*, offers information on five different categories of complementary and alternative treatments (CAT): herbal therapies, vitamin and dietary management, meditation and relaxation, neurofeedback, and sensory integration therapy. CAT are used widely in the USA; this chapter offers helpful basic guidelines and information, including references to books and Internet resources about CAT.

Chapter 11, *The Role of Play in Individual Psychotherapy from Childhood to Adolescence*, looks at how play may be used in the psychological treatment of children and adolescents. Specifically, I examine play therapy, a form of psychological treatment in which play is the central element for change and improvement. This chapter explains how play therapy helps and what it is like in practice.

Chapter 12, *Costs of Treatment: Money, Energy, and Time*, discusses the demands on you that can occur when your child is involved in treatment. I discuss issues to keep in mind if you need to advocate for your child with insurance companies or public service agencies.

The Appendix, *Self-help Resources*, gives many sources to help you further understand and help your child. I list general books about parenting and self-help books on specific disorders, as well as web sites for information and support. These resources will be useful in their own right and expand on the help you get if you do consult a professional. When you are better informed, you will be a better advocate for your child and a better participant in your child's treatment.

Why I wrote this book

This book grew out of my 30 years' experience as a practicing child psychiatrist. I have worked in clinics, schools, a residential program, and private practice. My work in these settings required me to draw upon my medical background and experience with medications, my training in normal and abnormal child development, and my training in a range of psychological treatments.

In each setting, a parent was typically the first person I had contact with about a child's problem. Parents always come with a bunch of questions. The particulars of those questions depended upon where they were on the path of helping a child with behavioral and emotional problems. If they were at the beginning of the path, the questions generally centered on trying to understand what was causing difficulty. Further along the path, the questions had to do with whether or not they could do something more to help and what kind of professional help might be needed or available. Some who had been on the path for a while had particular questions about the kinds of treatments that the child had been receiving and were wondering how to evaluate them and what other kinds of treatments might be considered. Wherever parents were on the path, they had their own emotional reactions to their child's struggles to cope with.

Because child psychiatrists have both medical and psychological knowledge and skills, they are sought after. Where I live, as in many parts of the USA, there are not enough child psychiatrists, or for that matter any kind of child mental health specialist, to provide timely help when it is needed. As a result, I receive many more phone calls from worried, distressed, and frustrated parents with questions about child mental health treatment than I can see in face-to-face appointments. So, I began to spend 15 to 20 minutes on the telephone trying to help the parent I could not see. I began to wonder if the kind of brief consultation that I was doing might be a model for a book.

The general organization of the book is based on the kinds of topics that came up in those telephone consultations. It has been expanded to include other areas that were of importance in my other contacts with parents. My goals in writing this book are:

- to respond to specific questions about what could be done to help a child
- to support the parents' efforts to make sense of a child's difficulties and help parents think more clearly about them
- to expand the parents' ideas about the causes and meaning of their child's symptoms so as to include both psychological and a medical/biological perspective
- to reduce the intensity of the parents' distress.

I hope that this book addresses many of your questions. Of course, it is not a substitute for an actual consultation with a mental health specialist.

A brief consultation

A woman who sounded in her thirties called about her seven-year-old daughter. Her little girl had been seen by a local child therapist. He thought that the girl needed to be seen by a child psychiatrist and might need medication for depression. This therapist

had a good reputation. I told the mother that although I had no time to see her and her daughter, I could talk with her and maybe give some recommendations. She seemed hesitant, but appreciative.

I assumed that the girl had symptoms severe enough to be diagnosed as depressed, like the therapist had said, but I also thought there was more to the story. Often when a child is depressed there has been a major loss or change in the family situation (such as a death, a recent divorce, or a parent's increased absence because of a new work schedule). Sometimes the changes seem less dramatic: the child might have started a new school, a younger sibling may have been born, an older sibling may have gone off to college, or a grade school teacher might have become ill and left the child's class.

I asked the mother when the symptoms had started. She said that her daughter had become acutely depressed ten days before. Her daughter seemed to cry "all the time," seemingly over very small and insignificant matters. She would regularly burst into tears at school and at home. The girl seemed inconsolable, and the mother felt overwhelmed by her daughter's distress.

She could not think of any significant changes in her daughter's life that had brought this on. I asked whether the daughter had ever behaved this way before; she said no, that her daughter was basically happy. However, she said that when her daughter was four years old she had shown some behaviors of concern that had led to sessions with a therapist. In the past, the girl had hardly ever complained about the pain of physical injury. Yet during the past week she would burst into tears over the smallest things and said she worried she would have to deal with injuries "my whole life." The mother also said that her daughter rarely referred to her feelings. Yet, the previous weekend, she had said she felt "ashamed" in school and seemed to feel guilty. Bursting into tears, she would ask her mother if she were going to punish her. The mother was jolted by this, since this was not her usual style with her daughter.

I asked about any major changes. The mother couldn't identify any, even after I went down a long list of possibilities. I wanted to assess how severe her daughter's "depression" was and if there were any suicidal thoughts or behaviors. There were none. Nor were there major disruptions in the child's sleep or appetite. I felt relieved that she was in no immediate danger. But this girl's emotional distress and her mother's worry were considerable.

I asked about the family situation. I learned that the mother was married and that her husband also worried about their daughter, their only child. I thought that it must be very difficult for this young mother, who had no older children to compare with this girl. She was emotionally invested in her daughter and the girl's distress stirred up a lot of distress in her. I wondered about the mother's experience of her daughter's suffering. She told me that despite doing all that she could do for her child, both verbally and physically, she felt quite helpless. Yet, she added, she was surprised when the little girl told the child therapist that her mommy was very helpful to her when she was

upset. The mother was concerned that despite doing all that she thought she could, she hadn't noticed any positive change in her daughter.

I asked the mother what she thought was causing her daughter's distress. She said she thought that her daughter was making some kind of change in her development, beginning to experience emotions and relationships in a new way. The little girl's mother believed her daughter was "knocked on her ass" by this upsurge of feelings.

I thought that the mother might be on target, but that she wanted her daughter to move more quickly through her distress than was possible. I noticed the contrast between the little girl's clear report of how helpful her mother was and the mother's experience of feeling helpless. I said that, from what she told me, her judgment of the situation seemed quite accurate. That is, her daughter was making some significant developmental changes and felt overwhelmed. I encouraged her to listen more to what her daughter said. I suggested that she might be more able to tolerate her daughter's distress knowing that she was helpful to her, even though not as helpful as she wanted to be.

We then turned to the issue of depression and treatment with medication. She expressed a worry about a "chemical imbalance" as underlying her daughter's difficulty. I explained that according to the formal psychiatric guidelines, a diagnosis of depression requires at least two weeks of symptoms, and this was only ten days. The reason for the two-week window is that many times the symptoms of depression are a passing response to some circumstance or change. Often the mood will improve as the individual adjusts to the change or as events improve. I thought that the child's mood was linked to some major steps in her development that were hard for her to accomplish and integrate. The girl would need time, support, and reassurance that her emotions "made sense." I encouraged the mother to return to the therapist with her daughter, at least for a few weeks. The therapist could help the little girl put words to, and organize, what she was going through. Therapy could also help the mother address her own concerns.

I gave her the name of a local child psychiatrist who might be able to see her more quickly for a face-to-face consultation. I said that unless something more had arisen than she reported, medication would probably not be prescribed immediately. Medication could be useful with intense emotional distress, whether related to a clear-cut diagnosis of depression or part of a developmental step. But it can take ten days to three weeks to take effect. I suggested that the most helpful thing to do right now was for the mother to continue to be kind and understanding. These responses would be helped along by frequent therapy sessions for them both, perhaps twice a week for the next three weeks.

I had three things in mind as I talked with this mother:

1. I wanted to help her think more clearly about what was happening within her daughter and draw upon her own natural good judgment.

2. I wanted her to see that she could decrease her daughter's distress.

3.   I wanted to help her better understand the use of medication.

A major part of the mother's ability to help her daughter came from their loving emotional attachment. The strength of their attachment encouraged hope and optimism in the daughter when her mother took steps to comfort and guide her through that difficult time. Thinking only in terms of a "chemical imbalance" that could be helped just through the use of medication belittled what she had to offer her daughter. With modest help from therapy, I thought that the mother would be the little girl's main support through a distressing and difficult life transition. I pointed out that her daughter's distress had been for a relatively brief time and the problem was neither life-threatening nor profoundly disruptive. The situation would likely respond to psychotherapeutic intervention. It seemed sensible to postpone starting medication.

However, I also knew there was a chance that the mother's help alone might not be enough. Sometimes a child's symptoms are so intense that, without the use of medication, a parent's abilities to help may be overwhelmed.

I considered that my taking a more wait-and-see approach to medication had to do with my distance from the immediate experience. If I had come into contact with the mother's earlier sense of helplessness and the little girl's distress, I might not have been as hesitant about using medication right away. However, I heard about the problems after some time had passed and the level of distress was not as pressing. I also heard about the mother's intuitive understanding of her daughter and the openness of the little girl to her mother's care. Because of these, I was able to help the mother see more clearly what she could offer her daughter that medication could not.

What I mean by "back on track"

This book is meant as a guide for you to help your child as he or she gets back on track toward health and wholeness. Regardless of the route, *you* are very important to the success of your child's journey. This book can help empower you to be the best helper you can be for your child.

Within each person, a remarkable force moves us toward wholeness and health. That force is involved when our bodies heal from illness or recover from injury. It also propels our mind/soul to rebound from psychological and emotional assaults. That force is strengthened by nurturing and diminished by neglect. But it exists in its own right, separate and distinct from what we do.

For parents, it is hard to balance two truths related to this force.

- We have tremendous power to nurture or diminish this self-healing force within our children, particularly when they are young.

- We have little power to direct or control that force, particularly as our children get older.

When you respect the positive force propelling your child's growth and development, you consider your child's autonomy, will, independence, hope, or choice. You understand that there are always elements within your child that strive towards wholeness, health, or "the right path." Sometimes you may feel like that force is not present in your child, especially if he or she persists in a course that seems filled with pain. But that positive force is always present, although it may be undermined by misunderstanding, confusion, disruptive emotions, or ignorance. When you are aware of that positive force, you are inclined to see your role more as one of helping, guiding, and nurturing than one of simply directing and determining.

This perspective may help you feel less burdened by unrealistically expecting that you can make your child feel or think a particular way. Even without this unrealistic burden, it is still very hard to guide, assist, and help your child develop into an individual able to care for him or herself, and for others. Thus, I chose to preface the title of the book with the phrase "*Help* Your Child or Teen Get." You cannot simply "get" your child back on track; you and others can only *help* your child with that task.

It is not always obvious what "back on track" means. Maybe your child is doing well, but then there are sudden upsetting changes. Your child may seem "off-track," and you just want to get him/her back to the earlier state of affairs. Many times that model works, but there are a few other times when it's more complicated.

First, what can *seem* to be "off-track"—with a lot of noise, heat, and sparks—may actually come from your child being right where he/she should be. For example, your child may actually be on-track, despite all the "heat and sparks," because he or she is moving through or into a new stage of development, such as entry into teenage years. Or your child may be involved in an unexpected life transition (such as adjusting to parental divorce) during which disruptive feelings (of fear, anger, and sadness) are normal.

Second, your child's "off-track" emotions or behavior may be a helpful signal to you that something is not working well within the family, your child's school setting, or social network. From this perspective, your child is "on-track" in showing his or her distress. So your child may be simultaneously off-track (in terms of a symptom) and on-track (in terms of communication).

Third, your child can *seem* to be doing well with few symptoms reflecting being "off-track." Yet years later, your adult son or daughter may tell you that that earlier time of life *was* one of being "off-track." At the time, you just didn't know about the depth of distress he/she was in.

So, most of the time it will be quite clear whether your child is on-track or off-track. But at other times there will be a lot of uncertainty, and the best you may be able to do is to tolerate the uncertainty, be thoughtful about it, and seek new understanding on your own or with the help of others.

During your child's adolescence, you may be especially unsure about whether he or she is "on" or "off" track. Teens, in contrast to younger children, have an increased say in their daily activities and direction. During this stage, your child's words or behavior may raise challenging questions: "Whose track/path is this, yours or mine?" "Where is this track/path going?" "Who's driving/leading this 'life'" and "How much control is possible, anyway?" These are complex and meaningful questions about existence that, as you know, return in a range of forms at various times throughout a person's life.

Despite these questions and the uncertainty, it falls to you to figure out if your child is "on" or "off" track, especially when your child is young and you might be regarded as the conductor/leader. As a loving and responsible parent, you try your best to help your child get back on the track that seems right. You try interventions on your own and may even consider getting professional help if things are not going as expected. That's what this book is about: what you can do and what professionals can do towards that goal of helping your child get back on track.

I hope you find that this book brings improved skills and new knowledge to thinking about the needs of your child and meeting them in the best way possible. It can be a guide to fresh ways of thinking about the meaning of your child's symptoms and to reacting to those symptoms. It is not a substitute for an evaluation by a child mental health clinician, but it can be a useful guide to the path you have to travel if you and your child do see a professional. I also hope that this book, with or without professional help, leads you to a deeper understanding of your child's emotional life and of your own.

Section I

PARENTS' INTERVENTIONS

The material in the following five chapters can be useful at any time. It can be particularly helpful before you seek professional help: before testing, before a diagnosis, and before entry into treatment. These chapters are particularly useful when you are:

- assessing the seriousness of what is going on with your child
- making sense of your child's symptoms
- figuring out what additional steps to take on your own to help your child
- struggling with your own emotional reactions.

Chapter 1

WHAT TO DO WHEN YOU THINK YOUR CHILD HAS A PROBLEM

This chapter is designed to help you cope with the questions and concerns that can come up when you first notice that your child is having an emotional or behavioral problem. One early question is whether what you are seeing is simply a passing phase of development requiring more of your attention and understanding, or whether professional consultation is needed.

Before addressing that question, this chapter offers you some useful perspectives for learning more about what is going on with your child. Through a simple question-and-answer format, the material in this chapter will help you be a better observer and listener. When you slow down to observe, listen, and think more carefully, your anxiety is likely to lessen. You will then be in a better position to bring to your child's problem more of your intuition, knowledge, and understanding. Also, you will be better able to evaluate the seriousness of your child's difficulties.

Questions and concerns typically come up when the problem a child is having is a new one for a parent. Since children are always changing, parents (particularly first-time parents) can encounter new problems quite a lot. Also, since each child's temperament, position in the family, and experiences in the world are different, each child presents distinctive challenges, even for the experienced parent. For these reasons, I consider parenting "on-the-job training."

From the child's perspective, growing up also is "on-the-job training." Children have to cope with the challenge that they are continually changing and coming up against new situations that they must master. They must constantly learn to:

- manage a changing body
- cope with changing emotions
- engage in new relationships
- take in new information about the world (see Chapter 3 for more detail about this).

In some of this chapter's questions and answers, I use the term "job" to refer to the tasks a child must become competent at as a part of growing up. This concept of having "jobs" can be helpful to a parent in several ways.

- You may find it easier to organize your efforts to figure out what is going on with your child.

- You may be able to bring more empathy to you and your child for the difficult work both of you are doing.

- You may find it easier to step back a bit from the pressure and worry that comes up when your child has a problem if you consider that what you have to do to help your child is a "job," one that takes time and effort to learn.

I remember how M. Scott Peck's statement in the first few pages of *The Road Less Traveled* (1998) that "life is hard" resonated deeply with me. I think this same kind of simple/honest statement can be made about the specific tasks of parenting and physical and mental development: raising children is hard work and growing up is hard work.

Another idea that underlies this chapter is the distinction between who your child is and the "problem" your child is having. The "problem" is a difficult, but most often time-limited and changeable, state that your child is in. Even if your child's problems are frequent or intense, he or she also functions well and feels untroubled at times. When trying to figure out what is going on with your child, keep in mind his or her more competent and capable sides. This is particularly helpful when you are under pressure from the more problematic sides. In doing this, you are then more apt to engage with your whole child, not just "the problem." You also are more likely to understand and help your child.

Organization of Chapter 1

The material in this chapter is presented in the form of questions and answers. The first seven questions address issues that can come up when parents begin to explore and evaluate a worrisome change that has been noticed in their child.

The next three questions address problems that arise in communication between parent and child: a parent feeling too distraught to cope well, a child who won't talk, and confusion about whether it's better to communicate by doing or saying something.

The last five questions address concerns that can come up with different parental responses to the worrisome change: punishment as a response to change; conflict between parents about seeking professional help; concerns about what treatment will mean; and concerns about safety while waiting for treatment.

Some of these questions may not apply to your particular situation. Information regarding particular difficulties for children of all ages can be found in Chapter 2, *The Red Flags: An Alphabetical List of Symptoms*. More specific information about difficulties for children at particular ages can be found in Chapter 3, *Disruptions in Development: The Whole Child*. Although virtually all problems or symptoms are found in both genders, I often use "he" or "she" to help the language flow.

Questions and answers

1. I think my child is having a problem. Now what?

When you begin to worry that your child has a problem, your focus might be either on behavior or emotions.

If your concern is about your child's behavior, your child is likely to have done something repeatedly, over a long period of time—something that you are annoyed, worried, or sad about. As in the examples below, your child's behavior may differ from how he has acted in the past. Or, if the behavior is not new, it may nevertheless concern you since it seems out of sync for a child of his particular age.

- Pamela's parents began to worry when their formerly sociable 11-year-old daughter spent excessive time in her bedroom alone, isolating herself from her family and her peers.

- James's parents began to worry about their adolescent son when he suddenly began skipping school.

- Frankie's mother began to worry about her fourth-grade son when she discovered that he was soiling himself and hiding his feces-stained underwear in the closet.

If your concern is about your child's emotions, usually your child has been feeling considerable anger, fear, or sadness for longer than usual.

- Sally's parents worried when, for no apparent reason, she began to be very frightened at night and when being dropped off at her elementary school.

- Barbara's father became concerned about his once even-tempered 13-year-old when she began to burst into tears easily for seemingly small reasons and to become enraged out of proportion to a situation.

Problem situations are most often a mixture of behavior and emotions. On first encounter we often just see one aspect of a problem. Just as we try to make out objects when we first enter a darkened room, we need time for our eyes to get adjusted to the new conditions before we can see more of what's present.

WHAT IF I'M MAINLY CONCERNED ABOUT MY CHILD'S BEHAVIOR?

If you, or someone who knows your child well, is concerned about how your child is behaving, think about your child's emotional experiences. All behavior has feelings and thoughts behind it. Sometimes it is fairly easy to figure out what the behavior may be expressing.

- Withdrawn and avoidant behavior may communicate feelings of anxiety or sadness.
- Repetitive behavior that involves destruction of property or injuring others may communicate anger and resentment.

Other times, figuring out what underlying feelings the behaviors are expressing may not be so easy. For example:

- troubling behaviors such as stealing, lying, substance abuse, impulsivity, compulsion or an eating disorder
- general traits such as controlling, demanding, and/or oppositional behavior.

Pamela's parents began to wonder if their daughter's withdrawal indicated that she might be feeling sad and depressed. James's parents began to wonder if their son's truancy was related to him worrying about something. Frankie's mother began to wonder if her son's return to soiling was connected to his immaturity and the fact that he frequently felt overwhelmed and confused by what was asked of him at home and school.

It can help to ask yourself "What feelings and thoughts *might* be leading my child to behave in this way?" Chapter 2 offers responses to this question in relation to specific behaviors.

WHAT IF I'M MAINLY CONCERNED ABOUT MY CHILD'S EMOTIONS?

You may notice that your child is experiencing emotional distress but you don't see much significance to it because your child's behavior is "okay." However, if you look at the behavior of your child in emotional turmoil, you may see that a problem exists. A depressed child may have a hidden eating disorder. An anxious and depressed child may be doing poorly in school, but not bringing home reports. An irritable and constantly angry child may be engaging in substance abuse unknown to his or her parents.

Sally's parents were concerned about her fear and sadness at home. They spoke with her teacher. She said that Sally had become quite bossy and demanding with her friend Lois. This had started after a third little girl had joined the class and Lois had spent time playing with the new girl instead of with Sally.

If it seems like just your child's feelings are problematic, look for behavioral changes also. This gives you an opportunity to help with some behavioral area of difficulty that goes together with your child's distressing feelings. Chapter 3 offers more discussion about specific emotional problems.

2. How do I know if my child's behavior and emotions are serious problems?

Let's look at why it is often so hard to judge this clearly.

DENIAL

It is hard to accept that your child, whom you love so much, is in emotional pain. You may want to minimize it or not even see it. This is particularly true when your child has emotional pain that you can acknowledge as present, but have difficulty understanding because it is so intense or has lasted so long.

> Mary's father understood why his daughter was sad when her best friend became best friends with someone else. He had thought, and hoped, that she would get over her sadness in a day or so. After a couple of days, he began to joke and tease her about the incident. She felt that he didn't "take seriously" how hurt, sad, and alone she felt.

You also may find it hard to accept your child's emotional pain altogether, particularly when its source seems completely mysterious or not significant.

> Sandra was happy that her adolescent daughter, Cathy, did not have a weight problem as she did. Sandra was proud of her adolescent daughter's slim and fit appearance. As a result, she was at first quite taken aback by how agitated and despairing Cathy got when she discovered on a visit to the doctor that she had gained a half pound in the preceding month. Sandra wondered why her daughter was making such a "fuss" about such a small weight gain. She was so pleased with her daughter's size that she didn't take in the fuller meaning of Cathy's emotional distress: Cathy was struggling with an eating disorder.

Sometimes, you don't see your child's emotional pain because you are so caught up in a painful situation in your own life that your child's distress is just too much to handle.

> Joe felt very guilty and ashamed that his marriage had ended in divorce. His guilt was so great he couldn't see that his son's depression about the divorce contributed to his not having enough emotional and physical energy to play basketball. Joe was upset his son didn't make the team. He thought his son was lazy, not depressed.

If you've had this kind of reaction, it's probably because you want to avoid further emotional pain. This wish gets in the way of fully realizing that your child's behavior or emotional state needs more attention. The more you acknowledge and take active steps to address the reality of your child's troubles, the more you are working towards diminishing your denial.

CHANGE

Your child is always growing and changing. In the midst of change, it can be hard to settle clearly on whether or not what you see is a normal part of change. This ongoing process of change adds to the challenge of parenting.

Many times, change is welcome and a source of relief. However, we may respond to an unexpected change with anxiety, worry, sadness, or anger. Even ordinary changes in life can be distressing. Our irritation with a situation will often come from our wish that a change hadn't taken place. This resistance to change makes it difficult to judge the importance of the change.

> Frances enjoyed being the mother of a young child. She loved being ever-present and watchful, offering hugs and comfort when needed. She told friends and family that she was very sad to see her "little boy" go off to school. When her son Joey seemed more anxious separating from her than she thought other boys did, she wondered if he was "too attached" to her. She questioned whether he was having a normal amount of anxiety around a new situation or was over-responding to her sadness and anxiety around their separation.

You may have similar uncertainty. Does your adolescent son's withdrawal into his room reflect a depression, or simply transient feelings of embarrassment in response to his changed body and changed interests? Is your daughter's repeated breaking of curfew the start of an oppositional disorder with underlying depression, or simply a response to increased social independence and less adult oversight?

Your child's behavior may also be influenced by other changes, such as marital conflict, separation, or divorce. If so, then your confusion may be compounded by worry that somehow you are to blame for the change your child has to cope with.

It is normal to feel confused and unclear about how to respond to new situations, particularly when you have not yet become familiar enough about a situation to know what to do. It takes time to deal well with change: to learn, reflect, become clearer about what you feel, and decide on the best response.

COMPLEXITY

Parent–child interactions become more complex as your child gets older. He is managing his emotions and relationships, as well as coping with the world around him. He has friendships and emotionally charged exchanges with people whom you may not even know. He has to make choices and figure out things all day long when he is not in your presence.

You, too, are struggling with similar tasks. For example, at work you interact with people who affect your emotions in different ways, and you too are deciding about how to deal with those people or your different tasks. Often it is hard to sort out whether your worry and irritation come from your own problems or your child's.

Richard returned home later than usual from a very demanding day. He wondered if he was cut out to be a manager and had felt his self-confidence quite shaken. Richard called his son Andrew to dinner one time. Andrew did not come. Richard then yelled at him to get off the phone. Andrew smashed down the phone and then sat sullenly at the dinner table. Richard thought that his son was being disrespectful of him and felt his confidence as a father shaken. Richard didn't know that his son was delaying getting off the phone because he was trying to work out a conflict with a peer, which had shaken his self-confidence. Richard's father was caught up in his own life complexity and thought that his son was simply being disrespectful. He didn't see that Andrew was caught up in his own separate challenges. At that moment, Richard didn't see his son struggling with self-confidence, in part because of his own self-confidence difficulties.

You and your child each have a range of separate experiences, thoughts, and feelings which can have little to do with what is immediately happening between you. It is hard to communicate when each of you has a lot going on. You will help yourself to deal better if you acknowledge how complex parent–child interactions can be. Chapter 4 offers some steps to help with this issue.

3. What simple guidelines will help me begin to understand the seriousness of my child's troubles?

Often, when you are trying to judge the seriousness of your child's troubles you are working at distinguishing between two paths: normal development and disorder/disruption.

In normal development, the symptoms are temporary, a part of growing up, and will resolve pretty much with your usual interventions.

In disorder/disruption, the symptoms are more long-lasting and may represent a pattern of behavior regarded as not normal. *Disorder* is a medical term that refers specifically to a group of symptoms that frequently occur together and have some common cause. For example, a depressive disorder may involve the symptoms of extreme sadness, difficulty sleeping, and an overload of self-criticism. *Disruption* is a more general term and usually means an interference with what is normal. These symptoms usually need more than your typical interventions. They need more of your time and attention—to understand and figure out how to be of help—than the ordinary day-to-day "bumps" in the road of growing up. Sometimes professional help is needed.

The following questions may help you decide whether the symptoms you observe are more likely to be normal development or disorder/disruption, and whether to consult a professional or not.

HOW FREQUENT IS THE SYMPTOM?

An occasional angry outburst that occurs once in six months over a big disappointment, such as the ending of a relationship, is normal. But tantrums which occur two or more times a week, particularly if over seemingly small matters, point toward disorder/disruption. Frequency, coupled with the symptom intensity, duration, or seriousness of consequence, provides a better guide to how soon to seek consultation than frequency of a symptom alone.

HOW INTENSE IS THE SYMPTOM?

Teenage annoyance and frustration with parents is common, but rage and anger with cursing, screaming, or threatening is unusual. Dieting is common, but a passionate and extreme preoccupation with food and body size raises significant concern. Intensity has a subjective element to it, with one person's tolerance for it higher or lower than another's. However, if you experience your child's symptom as intense, check out your perception with another adult.

HOW LONG-LASTING IS THE SYMPTOM?

Your child's crying spells, angry outbursts, or periods of intense worry that last many minutes are of less concern than similar behaviors that last for hours. Emotional states are usually of short duration. Compare the duration of your child's worrisome emotional state to other children of the same age, to your own, and to the duration of your child's other emotions.

WHAT ARE THE CONSEQUENCES OF THE SYMPTOM?

Distressing emotions or behavior may occasionally disrupt normal routine briefly. However, frequently disrupted attendance at school, much decreased peer contact, run-ins with the police, or dramatic changes in body appearance raise great concern that a disorder or major disruption is present and needs attention. When the consequence is more serious, even if not frequent, you ought to seek help more quickly.

HOW UNUSUAL OR "OUT OF CHARACTER" IS THE SYMPTOM?

A child who is outgoing and expressive and becomes more so is not especially of concern, but a child who goes from being quiet and shy to being very social and highly emotional would be.

Consultation is usually needed if the symptoms are frequent, quite intense, long-lasting and unusual, as well as socially, emotionally, or physically injurious. For more information about specific symptoms, and what you might do to help your child, see Chapter 2's list of "red flags." For a developmental perspective on your child and his or her difficulties, see Chapter 3.

4. How else can I distinguish between normal development and disorder/disruption?

Learn more about what is happening from your child's perspective. The best way is to talk with her. The type of "talking" that I mean is a time to listen. Ask her about what she is feeling. Show her that you are willing to take the time to listen to something that may be painful and difficult to hear. If you tend to tell your child what she is feeling, restrain yourself.

You may worry that you will cause more pain if you bring to the surface something painful that is inside your child. But often the opposite is true. A child who shares something painful with parents who understand and are accepting usually feels relief because she is validated. That relief far outweighs any brief increase in pain that may take place when the conversation begins.

However, talking about a painful experience may not work well because your child cannot express or reflect on her inner experience. Or she may not feel enough trust to be vulnerable. If so, use your child's nonverbal cues—observable details like facial expression, emotional tone in speech, bodily posture, and social interaction with others—to figure out what is going on. Such cues communicate helpful information about your child's emotional distress and may help you talk with her about what she is experiencing.

David's parents noticed that he was arguing more with his younger brother. He was more defiant with his mother and strongly opposed to joining the soccer team that he had been on the year before. He rarely laughed or smiled. At first his parents thought that their 12-year-old son was simply being cranky. But after a few months, they began to worry, even though he had not complained.

They decided to talk with him. They carefully chose the right time and place, making sure there was enough time and few distractions. They chose to talk to him when their annoyance and worry about his behavior were low.

They said, "David, you don't seem to enjoy things the way you used to." and "You've been angrier with your brother lately." When David heard his parents' concern and attention, expressed in a non-pressured way, he was willing to talk. He told them that it took him a long time to get to sleep every night because he was worrying about school the next year and how much he would have to do. He said he felt sad each time he took the bus home from his elementary school and wished he could be there for another year, like his younger brother.

His parents started to understand that he was feeling stress about the prospect of going into a larger school for seventh grade. Leaving the school that he had been in for six years was a big deal. Furthermore, his mother's increased work schedule left him feeling that he had to take on too much daily responsibility for himself. He also felt envious and angry with his younger brother, whom he believed got more attention than he did.

Like adulthood, childhood involves periods of confusion, misunderstanding, and conflict. Remember your own relevant experiences as a child. But also realize that your child's situation is inevitably different from how yours was. When you understand your child, you will then be more likely to find better ways to help him and know when professional involvement is necessary.

5. What challenges in the "job" of growing up can result in emotional and behavioral distress?

As I said earlier, growing up is hard work. Ordinary tasks, made up of different "jobs," can frequently give rise to emotional distress. Consider this example:

> Ten-year-old Johnny plays outside with his friends until his mother calls him in to have dinner. Usually he obeys and enters the house asking what's for dinner and what the other family members are doing. Sometimes, though, he enters looking as though he is about to cry, doesn't say much, and slumps into his chair. Every so often he may dawdle and have to be called several times. Occasionally he enters the house slamming the door, complains about having his game interrupted, and speaks harshly to his younger sister.
>
> In these last examples, distress is evident. His mother responds differently, depending upon her own state: (1) she may ignore his distress; (2) she may respond negatively, mainly out of her own distress, and become sad or angry herself, shifting the focus from his emotions to hers; (3) she may acknowledge his distress and try to learn what led to it.
>
> This third option is an example of discovering more about your child and the struggles he may be having with some aspect of his job: managing his body, emotions and relationships. Perhaps he was struggling with the frustration he can feel when an adult makes him stop something he is enjoying. This tests his ability to manage feelings of frustration and disappointment. Maybe he was stressed by leaving his friends who were continuing to play and wanted him to stay. This tests his ability to handle relationships.
>
> He had the ordinary but not simple task of taking his hungry and tired body inside his house, washing his hands, and eating. These were obviously tests of how well he could manage his body. He also had to deal with his mother's annoyance or disappointment if he didn't do what she wanted or as fast as she wanted. This again is a test of his ability to handle relationships.
>
> If his mother understood all that her son had to do when coming in for dinner, she might take his difficulties more lightly or not so personally. She might also be pleased about how well he did with managing his jobs. And she could then find it easier to help him discover better ways to cope with his jobs when he is distressed.

The next example is of an ordinary task, made up of different "jobs," which gave rise to behavioral distress. This distress expresses underlying emotions which the child was not able to talk about.

Sandra recently started junior high school. At first, her parents hadn't noticed any problems with the change. In order to make her breakfast and be ready for the school bus she had to get up earlier than she did in elementary school. This meant that she needed a new level of ability managing her body. After the first three weeks, she began to spend longer taking her morning shower and started missing the bus. Her parents' first response—reminding her and encouraging her to "move along or you'll miss the bus"—failed.

They recognized that this behavior was unusual for her. So they began by asking her how she felt about adjusting to a new school. They found out that she was frightened by the large number of classroom changes she had to make during the day (taking in new information about her world), unhappy that she had not made more friends (managing relationships), and ashamed to ask anyone for help (dealing with her emotions). Her fear, sadness, and shame came to the surface as she talked. Sandra had been afraid to bring these problems up with her parents earlier, thinking that she was old enough to deal with them by herself.

The discussions of symptoms in Chapters 2 and of disruptions in development in Chapter 3 offer more examples of the kinds of challenges in the job of growing up that can lead to distress.

6. What changes/stressors might make my child's "job" of growing up more difficult?

Your child may experience stress from any change in any job arena of life.

- Bodily changes. These occur most commonly with the changes of puberty, but also happen with medical illness.

- Changes in emotional experience. These occur when your child moves from pleasure in some activity to the disappointment of having to stop.

- Changes in relationships, as when a good friend moves away or a new teacher takes over the classroom.

- Changes taking place in the world around your child. These happen commonly when your child must move to a new apartment, house, or city, or take on some new sport or school challenge.

Being aware of your child's changing job tasks can help you be more aware of the stressors he may be experiencing. You can categorize changes and stressors along two dimensions.

1. Are they timely or untimely? This dimension captures the element of *expectation and surprise*. Unexpected changes/stressors are generally more difficult to deal with than those that are expected, and which allow for some preparation.

2. Are they external or internal? This dimension captures the element of *visible or invisible* to others. Changes/stressors not easily seen by others (like thoughts and feelings in reaction to external events) may be more difficult

for someone else to grasp. Therefore no one may offer help. Below, I elaborate on the four types of changes/stressors.

TIMELY CHANGES/STRESSORS

Timely changes are called developmental changes: they are challenges that all children go through at certain stages in the process of growing up. Examples include separation from mother, minor medical illnesses, going off to school, or conflict with loved ones.

Many children weather such changes/stressors relatively easily. But timely stressors can be quite disruptive and stressful to a sensitive child.

Timely changes/stressors, while difficult, will generally seem "normal." You most likely went through similar experiences as a child and can understand your child's reactions. However, you may still find these changes upsetting if your child responds to them differently than you did. Your child's reactions do not have to be just like your reactions in order to be considered "normal." Remembering this may help you be more accepting and supportive even if your child's reactions are more intense than yours were.

UNTIMELY CHANGES/STRESSORS

Untimely changes/stressors are not a regular everyday happening, which means that your child has no frame of reference to evaluate them. They include incidents like a serious medical illness in your child, serious physical or emotional impairment in yourself, or the death of someone close. Your child is more likely to feel stressed by untimely changes than by timely ones and consequently be in need of extra help and time to cope well with them.

These untimely changes can leave you feeling stressed and also insecure. For example, having your apparently healthy partner unexpectedly die of a heart attack would be overwhelming for you, as well as for your child. In such circumstances, you might not be able to help your child with the change as much as you would like. If family and personal resources are not enough to cope with untimely stressors, seek professional help.

EXTERNAL CHANGES/STRESSORS

External stressors are events that are visible. Examples would include moving to a new area, the birth of a sibling, parental divorce, or the loss or death of someone close. Other examples include physical illness in a parent or sibling, abusive treatment by someone who should be a protector, or repeated encounters with racist or sexist behavior in the world outside the family. External changes/stressors can be timely or untimely, either type may disrupt your child's sense of safety.

Table 1.1 Timely/untimely and external/internal changes

Timely changes/stressors	Untimely changes/stressors	
Weaning, change in routine	Parental divorce	
Sleeping alone	Disrupted living arrangements or frequent moves	
Toilet training	Accidents, exposure to violence	
Childhood illnesses	Life-threatening/serious illness in child or parent	
Starting day care/school	Alcohol and substance use	External changes/stressors, i.e. *events*, seen by others
Birth of a sibling	Racism and sexism	
Entering into competitive activities	Sexual abuse	
Bodily changes of puberty	Death of someone young (parent, sibling, friend)	
Death of someone elderly		
Emotional responses to timely external changes	Emotional responses to untimely external changes	Internal changes/stressors, i.e. *emotions*, seen and not seen by others
Emotional changes of puberty	Emotional responses provoked by physical illness	
	Emotional responses provoked by alcohol and substances	

Timely external change can be so familiar to you that you may not realize how stressful it is for your child. Common timely external changes, such as getting ready for school or settling down to bed at night, may involve a high degree of stress for some children. When not acknowledged, these times are often filled with conflict between parents and children. Timely external changes/stressors that are not acknowledged and validated (that are treated as if they were invisible) may be made more disruptive because of this non-response. Untimely (unexpected) external changes/stressors may be more disruptive than timely ones. When you are aware of how stressful an external change is for your child, you may allot more time for the change or give extra support.

INTERNAL CHANGES/STRESSORS

If an external change triggers unsettling thoughts and feelings for your child, then he or she also has to cope with an internal stressor. These sorts of internal reactions may be non-specific agitation or worry, or there may be detailed, exaggerated, and unrealistic fantasies together with intense emotions, such as panic, despair, rage, or utter humiliation. Sometimes these very strong internal responses outweigh whatever the external stress/change may be.

Emotional reactions are a natural and important way to make sense of an experience and let others know about it. But overly intense emotions may disrupt more than help. Throughout our whole life, we are working at balancing the positive effects of emotions with the potentially negative effects. If your child has intense emotional reactions to events, or a poor ability to maintain a balanced perspective, then she is likely to experience many internal stressors.

You can help your child learn to temper emotional reactions. When you spot the presence of internal stressors you will be better able to make sense of, cope with, and feel compassionate towards your child's struggle with the different jobs of growing up. You also realize more quickly that everyone is going through a hard time together. The following example makes clear the strong impact and importance that internal stressors can have for children and families.

> Eight-year-old Tommy was spending the night with some of his parents' friends because his father had to go to the hospital for a serious but not life-threatening procedure (*external and untimely stressor*). He was worried about his father. Because of his increased anxiety (*an internal change*), Tommy was shyer than usual with the children of his parents' friends. Reacting to his discomfort (*an external change for them*) the children teased Tommy (*external stressor*). He in turn became angry and more frightened (*internal stressors*). In response to that anger and fear, he began to imagine that his parents were going to abandon him and that his father was going to die (*more internal stressors*). He became even more frightened, angry, and sad.
>
> When his parents' friends saw that his emotional reaction to the teasing was so intense, they stepped in. They explained to their own children what Tommy was going through. They spoke to Tommy, noting that he seemed very worried. They reassured him that his father was not seriously ill and that he would see him the next day. They took steps to lessen Tommy's external and internal stressors.

In the preceding example, I emphasized the adults' intellectual understanding of change and stress. Their behavior more likely was guided by empathy. They understood Tommy's distress and also felt compassion for him. That compassion moved them to action.

7. What if I've seen no sudden changes in my child, but am concerned in general about the type of person he is "becoming"?

This common situation can be looked at in two different ways. First, your child's symptoms may have been present at a low level for a long time. As a result, you may have come to see these patterns as your child's way of being, rather than as expressions of a difficulty with some task in growing up. *Be careful not to interpret some specific problem as representing your child's total personality.*

Second, you may be responding to your child's temperament: an inborn pattern of reaction that influences behavioral and emotional responses. For example, your daughter may have a strong tendency to react with anxiety, shame, or shyness in new situations. She might have developed particular patterns of coping with emotions and relationships, which served her well when she was young. But as she gets older, these patterns could become a burden. For example, as a little girl she stayed very close to you as a way to feel safe. That pattern worked well. However, as she gets older, that pattern keeps her from having experiences by herself that would build her self-confidence.

On top of her temperamental patterns, you add your own patterns. For example, you might be somewhat overprotective when your daughter is distressed. Without realizing it, you encourage her to stay close to you in a new situation, as she seems more relaxed. Then you are both in a "dance" that perpetuates her earlier immature patterns. When you take this second perspective mentioned above, you will be able to think differently about "the person your daughter is becoming."

Your child's identity does not simply spring up within her. Rather, it is an outgrowth of her temperamental qualities and her relationship with you. This perspective can move you away from seeing your daughter as an unchanging "type" of person. It encourages you to see her as someone continually responding to the people around her and how she is treated by them. Your daughter may be temperamentally sensitive, but how you interact with her also influences her personality development. You and she will find that when things don't go well, it may be due simply to the ordinary struggles of growing up that happen between parent and child. And in those circumstances, it doesn't help to think of her behavior as due to the "type" of person she is.

> Michael's mother called me because her husband's psychotherapist had suggested, after hearing stories about the 14-year-old, that perhaps Michael should have a psychiatric evaluation. Michael's mother said that her son could be rigid, self-doubting, and avoidant of situations that his friends seemed to enter into easily. At that particular time she was not worried; he seemed to be relatively self-confident, engaged with others, and was open to new experiences. But she worried that perhaps the difficult times would return in one form or another and felt anxious about his future.
>
> She knew that she and her husband felt burdened and tired by the continued low-level struggle that they experienced in parenting Michael. She was also

aware that her worries about his future might distort her way of seeing him in the present. I noted that the difficult times with him seemed to come and go and that often it is hard to sort out how much turmoil has to do with the ordinary struggle of raising a child and how much is something that might warrant intervention. This is particularly difficult with a first child. I couldn't tell her which was which at that point.

However, I could say that if things were going well, it was not a good time to approach her son about a mental health evaluation. I explained that boys of his age tend to be embarrassed and resist the very idea of psychotherapy or medication, even when evident symptoms are present. Since Michael had no symptoms right now, it seemed to make sense to wait. She agreed.

I suggested that when they hit another difficult time, she could approach the issue from the perspective of family therapy. She might tell Michael that she and his father would like to work with him to find better ways to get through their frequent conflicts. She could add that they wanted to be the best parents they could be, and improving family communication would help with that. If they had some outside help, perhaps they could learn to communicate better.

Often, it is hard to remember that we cannot predict how life will go, or what life path our children will follow. We do our best on a day-to-day basis. Improving communication, sometimes with the help of a family therapist (see Chapters 7 and 8), can shift us from predicting future problems for a child to improving the present.

8. What if I'm so angry, frazzled, or scared that I want my child to "just stop it"?

Sometimes when you are having trouble with your own "jobs" (such as being a parent, holding down employment, or caring for yourself) you want your child to help *you* out. His emotional needs may weigh heavily upon you. You ask that he "just stop it!" Your longing for that is understandable. But usually, your child cannot "just stop." He is showing you with his strong emotions or problematic behavior that he is overwhelmed.

When you try to get him to "just stop it," you may add to his sense of isolation and aloneness with his problem and be bypassing an opportunity to learn about the details of his struggles and teach him how to deal better with his emotional distress. You teach your child by what you tell him to do with his distress and by what you show him in the way you handle your own distress.

But what if in a moment of your own intense distress, you demand that your child "just stop?" It happens; you're not a "bad parent." After all, parenting can be exhausting. Once you feel less stressed, let your child know that you had been feeling overwhelmed yourself and that your demand grew out of your own distress. Tell him that he deserves help with his difficulties, even if you can't always help him. Tell him that your goal is to understand his struggles and help him sort things out, even if you can't always live up to that goal.

If you find you often want your child to "just stop it," seek support from another adult who can help you get through those difficult times. If you are thinking about going to a professional, see Chapter 7, *Questions about Treatment: Who Are the Helpers and Where Are They?*

> Mary often began drinking when the stress from work, caring for her two children, and dealing with her own aged parents became too great. Her 14- and 11-year-old daughters sometimes became the object of her fury. This usually happened when they were worried and unhappy from their own struggles at school, interactions with friends, or the arguments between their divorced parents. Mary could not tolerate their misery and they could not tolerate her rages. A negative cycle of arguments and drinking would develop. Mary's yelling at them to "just stop it" simply drove them into their bedrooms and away from her. She later realized that whenever she drank, sending the children to stay with her sister was a protective break for them and her. This plan interrupted the negative cycles, helped her pay more attention to her drinking problem, and seek the professional help she needed.

Be aware of your own struggles and limits. See Chapter 4, step 10: "DO take care of your own physical and emotional needs," and Chapter 5, *Coping with Your Feelings When Your Child Suffers*.

9. What if I cannot talk with my daughter and she won't talk with me?

Children are often more sensitive to their parents' emotional states than parents themselves. You may communicate indirectly, as well as directly, to your child that you are overwhelmed. Either way, your child may withdraw in response to your pain or/and not share her own suffering in order to protect you. She might also feel overwhelmed by her own difficulties and assume that you would feel the same way or simply do not understand.

Remember that some period of blocked communication occurs in all parent–child relationships. When you notice a block that is new, seems significant and has lasted for a couple of weeks, consider seeking professional help. The guidelines mentioned in Question 3 (page 31) should influence how slowly or quickly you respond to the blocked communication.

If your child or adolescent balks at seeing a professional for help, try focusing on the problem in communication that is present in your relationship or in the family. Few children or adolescents will continue to oppose professional help if you show a willingness to explore your part of the communication difficulties. Remember, if your child resists family treatment, it may be because she wants to avoid exposure to distressing emotions. If you comment that whatever your child wants to avoid can be dealt with, acknowledge that you too have mixed feelings about treatment, and offer some incentive for after the meeting (like a stop for pizza on the way home) you will probably find much of the resistance to treatment disappearing. See Chapter 8 for more discussion on family therapy.

10. Once I think I understand my child, is it better to do *something* or say *something* to help her?

Often the most effective way to help involves *both* action and communication. There are times, especially with older children and adolescents, when we use words alone to clarify a situation, communicate about it, and bring about helpful change. Often, however, words are not enough. You may need to take some action to show your child what is needed to cope better. The younger your child the more some action is necessary. If you are taking action or want some action from your child, tell her why you are doing what you are doing. Also, speak in a way that shows that you empathize with her.

> Janet had a hard time focusing her attention, which contributed to her difficulty doing her homework. Usually she wanted to watch television with her parents before doing homework. Her father explained that because it took so much energy for her to focus and pay attention, he thought that school work should come first and television second. However, Janet found it difficult to sit at her desk and stop wandering into the TV room.
>
> Her father realized that the sound of the television was such a temptation to his daughter that neither his calm explanations nor his continued nagging helped. So he turned off the television and read. He did this to show that he respected her need for a quiet study environment. After a few months of this routine, Janet developed better study habits. She usually finished her homework before watching television, though she still needed reminders and encouragement.

A useful approach to a problem is to return to it later, even after several days. When emotions have cooled down, you will usually be able to talk about the conflict more calmly and act more thoughtfully. Children learn best, and parents teach best, in a calm state rather than an agitated one.

> In the previous example, Janet's father once became so upset that he yelled at his daughter, threatening that she would "never be able to handle high school" if her behavior didn't change. The next day, in a calmer mood, he returned to the incident and talked about his outburst, her behavior, and his worry. He apologized for unfairly yelling at her and told her that he now realized how difficult it was for her to study with the television on. After that talk, they arrived at a plan that felt acceptable to them both.

11. What if I understand my child's problems, but do not know how to make the changes needed?

This is a good time to seek help. There will come a time in your life, and your child's, when you clearly do not have all the answers. Don't get bogged down in your own disappointment and embarrassment. Others might make sense of difficulties and suggest ways to address problems when you can't. By reaching out you are showing your child how to work together with other people when difficulties seem too much to manage alone. See Chapters 7 to 11 for information on professional helpers and treatment, as well as the Appendix for self-help resources.

12. Can punishment lead to positive changes in my child and promote new ways of learning to cope?

Verbal or physical punishment tends to happen more from parental frustration than from a well-thought out teaching method. The essential component of punishment is to cause pain. This is usually done to stop a particular behavior or create fear of further punishment so as to prevent the behavior from happening again.

Verbal punishment can affect a child's sense of self negatively and impede good communication. Verbal punishment includes such things as name calling and making humiliating and belittling comments.

Physical punishment involves spanking and hitting. Such punishment mainly teaches something about what should *not* be done. At its worst, such punishment can become abuse. Simple physical punishment does not usually change a child's feelings, help her feel loved, or help her communicate better.

Imagine if you were engaged in on-the-job training and were periodically humiliated or physically punished for your mistakes. Imagine if your boss did not respectfully show you (in words and actions) when, where, and how you were mistaken, and you were not told what was required to do the job correctly. Your progress in learning the job would be slowed because of your worry and resentment about being humiliated or punished. You would be seriously confused with how to get around the difficulty and excessively preoccupied with doing things correctly. A good supervisor keeps in mind that supervisees do best when both sides are seen as working together, based on mutual respect, not fear. Parents, like good supervisors, generally do a better job at modifying a child's problematic behavior when fear is minimized, change is approached collaboratively, and a coaching or teaching style is used. See Chapter 2, *The Red Flags: An Alphabetical List of Symptoms* for new ways to understand and deal with specific problem behaviors.

So what kind of negative response (other than physical or verbal punishment) might be better? Having your child repair, replace, make amends or restitution, and lose privileges when appropriate, are all effective responses to misbehavior, especially when you stay lovingly aware of the child's viewpoint.

- A response that clearly teaches that breaking an object, rule, or limit leads to negative consequences.

- Your immediate disapproval for what has happened. This is best delivered in a clear, firm, and brief statement about the behavior: "Hitting is not the way to solve your problem with your brother!"

- Having your child repair or replace what was damaged.

- A fitting restriction of privilege or of freedom for a block of time might be a proper negative consequence for a violated rule or limit. Such consequences might also include an apology or making the situation better through some action.

Such sensible negative consequences, which do not involve physical punishment or belittlement, offer the best means to teach good behavior and produce long-term positive change.

The success of these interventions is also more likely to happen when your child understands why an apology and/or reparative action are needed. This gives you an opportunity to teach:

- fairness

- respect for others

- why there are rules for social conduct.

Of course, modeling such desired behavior in your relationship with your spouse, partner, and others is another way to teach your child such values.

> Angela was a high-spirited 13-year-old girl. She and a couple of friends had stolen some jewelry from a local store. Her parents discovered the jewelry. After questioning Angela, they learned where the jewelry had come from and that it had not been paid for. Angela had to return the jewelry in person and apologize for her behavior. She also had to offer to do some supervised work for the store owner in reparation for "injuring" the social contract of trust between herself and the store owner. Angela understood what her parents meant because she remembered how her father acted when he had not followed through on an agreed-upon plan he had made with his wife. He had accepted responsibility for the lapse in his own behavior, apologized, and made amends.

Imposing negative consequences, especially those that make sense, are a much more effective way of getting the kind of proper behavior desired than simple punishment aimed at causing pain to change behavior.

13. I want to get professional help for my son, but my husband thinks he is "just being a boy" and that I'm making too much of it. What should I do?

When parents disagree that a problem exists for a child, it is commonly the father who takes the position of there being "no problem." Under such circumstances, I encourage the father (or the mother if she takes that position) to attend the first consultation. At the very least, this gives that parent a chance to offer a different view. Sometimes it turns out that the difficulty is not primarily with the child, but mostly with parent–child interactions or parental expectations.

When the problem needs to be addressed directly with the child, I encourage both parents to take part as much as possible. If one parent refuses to participate, I will work with the parent who agrees. I let the non-participating parent know that he/she is welcome to take part in the treatment process at any time.

Occasionally the "split" between parents about whether there is a problem reflects the stress on both adults of having a child with problems. Parents may take such opposite positions because they have different styles of managing the hurt, fear, and disappointment about their child's difficulties. In the face of disturbing emotions, one parent may be more likely to minimize the difficulties and the other may be more likely to magnify the difficulties. Under these kinds of circumstances, a marital relationship can become quite strained. Seeking help, working on the difficulties, and making progress can reduce the strain on the marriage.

14. If I do seek a professional consultation, does that mean my child will go on medication and be in treatment for a long time?

Your first few meetings with a child mental health professional will usually help shed light on the nature of your child's problem, figure out what is contributing to your child's problem, identify your child's strengths, and develop a plan.

If your child is young, the consultation or treatment may primarily involve the parents. If your child is pre-adolescent or older, then he or she most likely will be actively involved in the consultation and treatment.

Treatment may be limited to a few meetings or to much more; it is quite variable. Medication may be used as part of treatment, but most children who are referred for evaluation and treatment to a child mental health specialist do not go on medication.

For much more detailed information about the particulars of child mental health treatment, please see Chapters 8 to 11. Chapters 8 and 11 focus on psychotherapy, Chapter 9 on medication, and Chapter 10 on alternative treatments. Chapters 8 and 9 each have a "frequently asked questions" section in addition to the section that has specific information about the particular treatment.

15. What if I'm waiting for an appointment with a specialist, but I am worried about my child's safety and mine?

Such a situation can be frightening. Your parental role to protect your child or adolescent may be pushed to the limit. You may be unsure about whether you can keep your son or daughter safe.

Most communities have mental health emergency staff available 24 hours every day. The staff may be part of your local mental health clinic or connected with the emergency room of your local hospital. If you decide that you cannot keep your suicidal or self-destructive child safe, or that you yourself are not safe from harm by your child, call for help.

Typically, it makes sense first to call the mental health crisis unit or emergency room of your hospital to speak with staff about the particular situation. But if the situation is dire, your first call may need to be to your local police or 911. The police can transport your child or adolescent safely to the crisis unit or emergency room for evaluation. See Chapter 7 for more information about mental health emergency service agencies.

In reading this chapter, you may have learned:

- a sensible approach to common questions that can come up when you first notice something not right with your child
- suggestions that can help you think more clearly and calmly about the trouble
- ideas for how to interact better with your son or daughter about the trouble
- answers to common early questions around seeking professional consultation.

In Chapter 2, I am more specific about particular behaviors or emotions that have caught your attention—what I call "the red flags."

Reference

Scott Peck, M.D. (1998) *The Road Less Traveled: A New Psychology of Love, Traditional Values and Spiritual Growth*. Old Tappan, New Jersey: Touchstone Books.

Chapter 2

THE RED FLAGS:
AN ALPHABETICAL LIST
OF SYMPTOMS

Contents

The goal of this chapter is to help you better understand and respond to your child's "red flags"—the symptoms that call for your immediate attention and provoke worry and preoccupation. Your intense concern and anxiety occurs mainly because what you are dealing with feels quite unknown. This chapter will help you think more clearly about what's causing the "red flag," its level of seriousness, and how to respond to it.

It can be difficult to understand the cause of a "red flag" for several reasons. The causes of symptoms can be varied:

- *biological* causes: a sensitivity or impairment at the chemical and physical level

- *psychological* causes: a sensitivity or impairment at the level of emotions or thoughts

- *developmental* causes: a delay or problem with some stage or "job" of growing up: managing the body; coping and dealing with compelling emotions and thoughts; engaging in relationships; and taking in information about the world (see Chapter 3 for a more thorough discussion of the developmental perspective)

- *social* causes: stress or lack of support coming from family, friends, or community.

- Several causes can contribute simultaneously to one symptom.

- The same symptom can come from different combinations of causes.

It can be difficult to gauge the seriousness of a "red flag" for several reasons.

- There is almost no behavior or mood that *always* indicates a disturbance and the need for treatment.

- It is hard to predict the long-term impact of the symptoms on your child's future mental health, even if the current seriousness is apparent.

- Children are constantly changing, so it is hard to gauge the seriousness of a symptom. Behavior that is common in a young child is often seen as disordered in an older child. For example, young children often distort reality and make up wild stories as if they were true, but a teenager showing this same behavior may be regarded as highly immature or experiencing a serious disturbance.

It can be difficult to gauge how to respond to a "red flag" for several reasons:

- In our worry, confusion, and wish to help, we often rush to give the symptom only one meaning or cause.

- Oversimplifying the meaning of a symptom leads to oversimplifying the kind of treatment needed.

For example, there is currently much pressure to identify symptoms such as depression as indicators of some kind of particular "chemical imbalance." This view addresses the biological causes and seems to point to a biological (medicine) intervention. This level of analysis can be helpful, yet neglects the psychological factors (how your child views himself and others), social factors, and life circumstances (like the stresses or supports present in work or school, and in family, friend, and love relationships). These psychological and social factors can contribute significantly to depression and should be treated with psychological or social interventions.

It is also difficult to gauge how to respond to a "red flag" since one must judge whether developmental causes are involved.

- Is this symptom a part of normal development/life or an actual disorder?

- If a disorder, can normal parental love, understanding, guidance, and action alone provide the cure?

- Is professional consultation and intervention needed?

The material in this chapter will help you with these questions as they apply to individual symptoms. Also reconsider what I discussed in Chapter 1: if the symptom is very frequent, quite intense, long-lasting, widespread, or socially, emotionally, or physically injurious, then professional consultation is warranted.

Although there is much information about medication in Chapter 9, I'll close out this introduction with a few words addressing a question that frequently comes up for parents. How can medication help behavioral problems and troubling emotional states which are rooted in the child's psychology and inner life?

It's true that research scientists understand how certain medications affect specific areas and chemicals in the brain. Yet we actually know very little about how or why these medications are effective. What we do know is that the right medication can help an individual better modulate (keep in balance) emotions, thoughts, and attention. Medications help us to use our best coping skills, rather than respond to a situation in ways that may be too emotional, highly detached, overly self-centered, or very impulsive. When a child can handle his inner responses better, he can cope with stressful situations better, behave more appropriately, and communicate more effectively with others.

Organization of Chapter 2

In this chapter, I address an alphabetical list of symptoms. For each I offer:

- a psychological point of view to help you better understand your child's inner experience—this may include a developmental perspective, i.e. how your child's stage of growth and maturity contributes to the symptom

- a medical/psychiatric or management perspective for the more troubling "red flags"

- A "Possible intervention," which is a kind of psychological first aid. This can offer you new ways to interact with and assist your child, although it may only be a part of what is needed. Professional treatment, medication, and psychotherapy, may also come up in a "Possible intervention."

The symptoms listed below, unless otherwise specified, are not gender-specific. However, to make the discussion as clear as possible, I alternate between describing a child as male or female. Words that are in bold type refer to other topics in the red flags list.

The symptoms

Aggressiveness: Aggressiveness is present in a child who is excessively forceful in his interactions with others. It may show up when he is pushy, grabby, threatening, or behaving in an excessively rough way. Increased aggressiveness may accompany almost any emotional disorder, such as depression or panic attacks.

Aggressiveness may exist because of a chronic feeling of anger. The trigger has not been adequately recognized, acknowledged, or addressed by the important adults in a child's life. Perhaps a child does not even know the causes of his anger. He may then be aggressive towards someone or something that relates only indirectly to the actual cause of his anger.

If your child shows aggressiveness that is more than normal for a child of his age, then his abilities for coping with anger may be overwhelmed and he may have a lot of anger. Or your child may have a normal level of anger but has not developed age-appropriate ability to cope with, and communicate, his anger.

Possible intervention: see **Anger**

Anger: Anger is a normal human feeling that communicates your child's distress and energizes him to do something about it. It becomes a problem if it flares up too quickly, or intensely, or is improperly expressed.

If your child is quick to anger, that means that she reacts immediately, or over-reacts, to whatever triggers distress. This may indicate a low tolerance for frustration. Triggers can include things that are immediately irritating or depriving of pleasure, such as being asked to turn off the television set or get off the telephone. Or these may be long-lasting irritants that underlie a low flash point, such as an unfulfilled wish to be an only child or for divorced parents to reconcile.

Your child may direct her anger at the person seen as denying her desires. For example, she may yell at you if you ask her to care for a sibling or to do her homework. Or she may direct her anger at someone only indirectly connected with the distress. For example, she may yell at a new step-parent (anger about the divorce), the unwanted sibling (anger at parents for decreased attention), or even an innocent bystander (anger at family member or friend). Finally, she may direct her anger at anything that represents the source of the distress: a school notebook, a broken bicycle, or a "no skateboarding" sign. The behavior and words may be appropriate for a child her age. Or they may not be.

Frequently, anger is accompanied by other feelings like shame, fear, and sadness. These feelings may be obvious or may be overshadowed and hidden by anger. These other feelings may also contribute to the intensity of the anger your child expresses. For example, your child may primarily be very sad, although also somewhat angry, about losing something she deeply wanted. She may be unable to handle the complexity of her inner experience; as a result, her intense sorrow may be expressed simply as anger. The same may be true of fear. Anger may cover over unacknowledged fear.

Angry feelings are a part of life. But anger that is overly intense, frequent, long-lasting, or that is expressed in destructive and injurious ways, must be dealt with. Persistent, excessive, or injurious expressions of anger may be linked to specific disorders, such as **Depression** or **Mood swings**.

Possible intervention: Start by talking calmly with your child about the ways that her anger is a problem.

- Try to identify specific stresses she is dealing with. Talk about them and acknowledge them to help her feel not so alone with her misery.

- In a situation of some life-altering change or major event (such as a divorce), actively listen for feelings of shame, fear, or sadness that your child needs help identifying and coping with.

- Look for ways to improve your child's tolerance of distress. Help her list ways to comfort herself when distressed or develop interests that will increase good feelings about herself.

- Encourage her to use words, rather than actions, to express her anger.

- Encourage her to practise expressing thoughts and feelings regularly in a calm and clear way, rather than in brief, loud, vengeful outbursts.

- If the situation does not improve, seek professional intervention.

Anxiety: Anxiety that comes and goes is normal. When mild or moderate, anxiety raises a child's level of alertness for dealing with new, demanding, or dangerous situations. However, anxiety may be elevated to the level of panic and be so persistent that it interferes with everyday life. Your child's high level of anxiety may show up in a range of behaviors. Most symptoms have some element of anxiety, so refer to the specific symptom that seems to accompany the anxiety: for example **Obsessions, Compulsions, School avoidance**, etc.

Possible intervention: You must walk the line between two different approaches to anxiety. First, help your child tolerate anxiety and learn that he can put up with it and that it passes. Second, help your child move away from anxiety through constructive distractions and use of coping mechanisms.

- Help your child not feel so alone. If he experiences your empathy for what he's going through, he may feel significantly better.

- Help him make sense of what he is experiencing by identifying anxiety as a normal emotion that each person must learn to cope with, and learn what triggers it (see Chapter 4, step 5: "Do help your child to confront fear" and see Chapter 6).

- Help your child learn a range of relaxation techniques that have been developed by psychologists. There are many audiotapes and CDs for learning progressive relaxation and mindfulness. See the Appendix for specific references.

- If your child's anxiety, or the accompanying symptoms, seem unusually intense or interfere with relationships or work, seek professional consultation.

- Psychotherapy, with elements of cognitive behavioral therapy (see Chapter 8), helps by identifying and challenging irrational thoughts that increase anxiety.

- At times, medication can dramatically reduce your child's disabling anxiety.

Avoidant behavior: Your child may deal with inner distress by staying away from the places and situations that seem to trigger her agony. This avoidance may be limited to particular situations (like school) or may be more general (like avoiding any new people or places). An increase in avoidant behavior may indicate a high level of **Anxiety** or an underlying **Depression**. You may also have noticed a pattern of behavior that includes **Shyness** and **Rigidity**. See these highlighted symptoms, as well as **School avoidance**.

Possible intervention: Your child's distress may be most clear when she runs into the situation she wants to avoid. But her general level of inner anguish may also be high.

- Communicate to her that you understand her distress but that you also believe she can handle the events that seem so difficult.

- Consider accompanying her to particular situations she wants to avoid, to help her confront her fear successfully.

- Psychotherapy, with or without medication, can help diminish the intensity of her distress and address the underlying difficulty.

Bedwetting: see **Wetting**

Bullying: Bullying is defined as any aggressive behavior that 1. has the aim of causing injury, upset, and/or humiliation, 2. is repetitive, and 3. occurs between individuals with an unequal balance of power. Bullying may involve open attacks (like hitting or verbal abuse) or may be more secretive (with exclusion, isolation, and the spreading of rumors and lies). Both girls and boys can be a perpetrator or a target of bullying.

Most children who are bullied are shy, quiet, have few friends, and are worried about being hurt emotionally or physically. Long-term consequences of being bullied may be depression and low self-esteem.

Most children who bully need power and dominance, are inclined to have a hostile attitude towards others (peers or authority figures), and frequently break rules. But some bullies may be successful at school and have no obvious conduct problems. If the behavior is left unaddressed, the bully may develop serious adult antisocial behavior.

Bullying affects children immediately involved and those who are bystanders. Bullying in social environments (class, school, or other social settings) undermines the general feeling of safety and mutual respect.

Depression can be associated with being bullied; **Oppositional behavior** can be associated with bullying.

Possible intervention: If your child is doing the bullying, respond quickly and firmly:

- Tell him, "Bullying is not acceptable behavior."
- Tell him there will be specific non-physical and non-belittling negative consequences (such as losing privileges or receiving penalties) if he continues to bully.
- Deliver this information in a concerned and caring manner.
- If bullying is taking place mostly at school, contact the teachers to get their help. This will improve teacher awareness regarding bullying and back up their efforts to create a safe school environment.
- If bullying is taking place mostly in the neighborhood, work with other parents.
- Provide positive rewards for not bullying.

If your child is the object of bullying, also respond quickly and firmly:

- Tell your child and other adults: "Bullying is unacceptable, and I will see that it comes to an end."
- If the bullying is taking place mostly at school, contact the teachers to let them know of the need to address this problem immediately.
- If bullying is taking place mostly in the neighborhood, contact other parents, who normally will not want their child to engage in such behavior. Contact parents whose children are doing the bullying as well as those who may be bystanders or victims.
- Give your child a safe forum in which to express how he feels about the bullying, and be able to express limits for what behavior he will accept.

- Support your child in asserting his rights firmly and forcefully, and in learning how to get effective help to stop the bullying.

- Do this in a respectful, non-blaming, and non-reproachful manner. This will help the parents of the bullies, and will help encourage other parents to share their awareness or concerns about the problem. Adults must work together to provide appropriate neighborhood communication and supervision.

Much of the preceding material is drawn from *Bullying at school: What We Know and What We Can Do (Understanding Children's Worlds)* (1993) by Dan Olweus (see Appendix, "specific problem/symptom focused books").

Cheating: Episodes of cheating indicate that the child has not yet developed a socially acceptable balance between two opposite impulses: the desire to be singled out as special and the desire to share and feel connected to others.

Cheating happens when a child's need to win is so powerful that it overcomes his normal desire for cooperation and fairness. Some children may cheat because they cannot tolerate the disappointment that comes with losing. The loss, which feels intensely like a personal failure, may be connected to some other sense of inadequacy that exists in a more significant area of life. For example, the child may fear that someone she loves profoundly disapproves of her and she can't figure out how to win that love. Cheating can block your child from developing solid relationships and a healthy sense of self-esteem.

Possible intervention:

- Help your child identify what she is good at and support her natural desire to be connected to peers.

- Point out that learning to cope with the difficult feelings connected with losing is everyone's job in growing up.

- Encourage her to get involved in a team sport or in games and activities that have the goal of winning but require that your child follows rules and cooperates with others. Most often these are activities in which the team is "the winner" and all participate.

- Encourage her to get involved in activities that don't involve winning or losing (i.e. community activities). This may provide a temporary relief from her inner conflict and give your child an unconflicted way for her to increase her self-esteem.

Clinginess: Your child may cling to you if he is scared of being alone or injured. His worry about being alone may be connected to a worry about being abandoned; worry about injury may be connected to feeling vulnerable and scared that the protective parent may disappear. See **Separation anxiety**.

Possible intervention: There is always conflict underlying your child's clinging. His desire to be independent is temporarily overwhelmed by his fear and desire for protection.

- View this situation as temporary, rather then a lasting character trait.
- Validate his distress and remind him that you know he wants to be more independent.
- Agree to work together to decrease his fear.
- Support his independence by noting his accomplishments in that direction.
- Communicate your confidence in his ability to learn to tolerate and cope with his fear.

Compulsions: Some degree of compulsive behavior is normal, especially during middle childhood from seven to ten years. But if your child engages in repetitive driven behaviors that are frequent, long-lasting, seriously interfering with social functioning, and reflecting severe internal distress, this is a problem, and she may be formally diagnosed with obsessive–compulsive disorder.

"Obsessive" indicates the presence of repetitive thoughts or ideas that cause a lot of anxiety. I discuss these under **Obsessions**.

"Compulsive" means that your child does repetitive actions or rituals, like frequent hand-washing, non-stop counting, or endlessly collecting objects. From a psychological perspective, this behavior is understood as action to get rid of the anxiety and fear associated with obsessive thoughts. The compulsive behaviors often seem irrational to those around your child and usually to your child herself. This is especially so when your child thinks the rituals will magically protect her against something she dreads. The sense of dread may be described as only a feeling or may be accompanied by specific thoughts and ideas.

Driven by intense worry, your child may feel she has no choice about performing these actions. Because she has little distance, or perhaps no conscious awareness of her emotions, she cannot separate her feelings of terror from the actions she takes to eliminate those feelings. A common compulsion, such as the superstition of "knocking on wood" to ward off something feared, has some of the emotional quality of such rituals. But the *intensity* of the feeling that is part of compulsions is not usually present in everyday superstitions.

Possible intervention:

- For compulsions that are mild and not terribly disruptive, gently support your child to confront her fear of not doing the ritual.
- Encourage her to stop performing the behavior for as long as possible, tolerate the anxiety, and put into words whatever is frightening her.

- Help her think about, identify, and find more effective ways to understand and cope with situations that trigger her fear.

- Seek cognitive therapy (see Chapter 8) to help your child learn to cope with her anxiety better and develop a graded program to stop the compulsive behavior progressively.

- For compulsions that are very intense and disruptive, medication can help eliminate them.

Cross-gender dressing: see **Gender identity confusion**

Crying: Crying is an automatic call for help that communicates sadness and distress. It can also accompany anger or fear. The crying and sadness are usually a response to a loss (real or imagined). Sometimes the importance of the loss may not make sense to another person. Whether or not the loss makes sense to you, your child's emotions need to be acknowledged and respected. Often, crying is a healthy response and indicates that your child has begun to accept the reality of the loss. Sometimes, the absence of crying indicates that your child is trying to avoid a fuller acceptance of a painful reality.

Crying may be intense or prolonged. Crying that seems excessive in an adolescent may be appropriate in a young child or just a function of normal temperamental variation at any age. But it also may indicate some disorder, such as **Depression**.

Possible intervention: Always respond to crying with sympathy and comforting. Expressing sympathy does not mean that you have to comply with your child's desire for a particular way to feel relief.

- Do not tease or allow siblings to do so.

- Acknowledge and validate your child's feelings to help him begin to accept that things are not how he wishes.

- It is not always helpful to take action, particularly when the crying is part of a normal process of adjusting to a loss. Doing something to interrupt the normal process of sorrow or grief may be a disservice to a child's ability to develop the capacity to cope well with loss.

Delusions: Delusional thinking distorts some aspect of reality. If your child is experiencing this kind of thinking, you may have a hard time understanding some of his actions and/or reasons for those actions. For example, your son may believe that the teachers want him to fail. He may believe that they are arranging the examinations in a manner for him to fail and decide not to go to school. This explanation is not easily changed; he may fully view it as "reality." This is in contrast to the made-up story of a younger child who just is fantasizing and knows that the story is not real. Delusional explanations are more commonly found in older children and adolescents.

From a psychological perspective, your child may have delusional thinking when he feels vulnerable, unprotected, and overwhelmed by extremely distressing emotions (see **Fantasizing**).

Possible intervention: Delusions are thoughts that are not easily changed by reasoning. But you may help your child by grasping the depth of his distress.

- Help your child talk about his painful feelings.

- Show empathy for his distress.

- Seek professional consultation to figure out other steps to help diminish this way of coping/thinking as well as unknown sources of his distress.

- Medication may help your child by settling deeply turbulent emotions, enabling clearer thinking about what's real and what is not, and allowing psychotherapy to be more effective.

Depression: Depression is an ongoing state of painful sadness. In contrast to simple sadness, the sadness of depression often goes along with frequent crying, ongoing anger, intense shame and guilt, and disruptions in sleep and appetite.

Your child may become depressed in reaction to a change or loss in his life that he experiences as permanent, intolerable, and irresolvable. This change or loss might be obvious (such as the loss of a beloved home or friendship because of a family move), or not obvious (such as the loss of a sense of competence or independence).

Most often the trigger is a combination of these two qualities: it is a real event that has important internal meanings. Your depressed child feels stuck, hopeless, and often personally responsible for the situation. At their most extreme intensity, these feelings may occur together with suicidal thoughts (see **Suicidality**).

Possible intervention:

- Acknowledge the loss and help your child find ways to talk about and respond to this loss. This may reduce the intensity of her depression.

- If her distress and the disruption in her functioning are intense, consider professional help.

- Seek individual or family therapy to help you and your child identify what the change or loss may be and to find better ways to cope.

- Although medication can be very helpful, do not use it as the only intervention (see Chapter 9 under "Pharmacotherapy: frequently asked questions," number 2).

Disobedience: Usually children show some degree of rebellion as a way to express their individuality and development towards independence. But if your child regularly defies your authority or does not comply, you probably have cause for concern.

He may be copying the behavior of an adult who is important to him, seeking his favor. For instance, your child may see his father typically respond negatively to others, such as his teachers. He may model himself on his father and behave in ways that seem to fulfill his father's expectations. Or he may harbor anger toward important authority figures on his own.

Often a disobedient child has a hard time tolerating negative emotions (anger, sadness, shame, fear) associated with not getting things his way. Chronically disobedient children may also have a high level of **Impulsivity**: they tend to respond immediately, and without reflection, to strong emotions.

Possible intervention: Try to gauge whether this behavior has been present for just a little while or is a major ongoing problem with disobedience and disruption in many situations.

- If the behavior is limited to the family setting, seek family therapy if your child seems to be modeling the behavior of older family members.

- If your child is disobedient in many settings, then individual therapy, in addition to family work, may be helpful.

- Medication may be helpful if extremely strong emotions, such as intense **Anger** or **Depression**, or **Impulsivity** are major factors. (See Chapter 9, "How medications/chemicals affect behavior," p. 213.)

Drug use: An adolescent may begin to experiment with drugs or alcohol for many reasons. She may seek to alter her thinking or emotional state. Or she may be responding to the social environment, seeking peer support and bonding. For many, it stays at the level of joining in at a party. For others, it progresses to more frequent weekday usage. A child who is highly prone to peer pressure and feeling alienated from family is vulnerable to being a high frequency user.

Many young people who become involved with regular substance usage are trying to "treat" their emotional distress. Ironically, the more your child turns to drugs to mute and contain her feelings, the more difficult it is for her to develop age-appropriate ways to deal with her emotional life. The more frequently a child uses drugs, the greater the risk to physical safety and to emotional and psychological well-being.

Possible intervention:

- Be clear about your own values regarding illicit or excessive use of substances.

- Although drug use is widespread, it usually has a particular meaning for each child. Ask yourself: Why has my child chosen this path? What distressing emotion or situation is my child escaping from or trying to cope with in this way?

- If you experimented with drugs in your past, go back over that experience from your adult viewpoint and talk with your child about it.

- Have this conversation authentically. Be truthful about your own past behavior and your current views of that behavior. Be honest about the allure of substance use that you may have felt, or may still feel, even if you are not using now. Distortion or hypocrisy on your part will only make things more confusing.

- Consider family therapy and participation in a drug treatment program. A program can help you and your child learn appropriate and constructive responses to your child's substance usage or abuse.

- Since underlying depression or other emotional difficulties are often a part of the substance abuse problem, psychological therapy and medication treatment may be necessary.

- If you or your spouse currently use drugs or are alcoholic, it will be harder to discuss and address your child's difficulty.

Eating disorders: Eating disorders happen predominantly in females, although they now occur more frequently in boys than 15 years ago. An eating disorder can take different forms. Your child may diet or exercise excessively because of a worry that her body is getting too big. She may stuff herself with food and then secretly vomit it up.

She may have an impaired ability to tolerate and talk about her distressing emotions. She is trying desperately to cope with a naturally complex emotional life by simplifying it through focusing on and controlling one narrow arena: her food and her body. Unfortunately, such narrow preoccupations keep her from developing better ways to cope with her emotions, which would lead to a more positive sense of self and more satisfying relationships with others.

Possible intervention: Eating disorders are prevalent. Sometimes they are fleetingly present, but keep in mind that this disorder can be serious, even life-threatening.

- Do not wait for a more extreme state to develop or for your child to bring up the topic herself before you consider treatment.

- If other members of the family have unusual eating patterns, ask your child for her perspective on this.

- Consult your family physician or pediatrician, who can give an objective judgment of what your child's proper weight should be and how to identify and manage this problem medically. The doctor can attend to and treat the potentially dangerous physical effects of an eating disorder.

- Seek family therapy, especially within one year of the onset of symptoms, to address problems in communication, especially of emotionally charged issues, that often intensify with the presence of an eating disorder.

- Consider an eating disorder program, a 12 step program like Overeaters Anonymous, along with individual therapy.
- If depression or anxiety is a big part of this problem consider medication (see Chapter 3 on Adolescents: disruption of bodily routine, page 114).

Encopresis: see **Soiling**

Envy: Envy is a normal though painful emotion. It is a mix of desire, shame, anger, and fear. It becomes a problem only when it is persistent, intense, and it crowds out more positive emotions. Persistent envy can lead to poor peer relationships and chronic feelings of deprivation or inadequacy.

Your child's envy may be directed toward someone else's possessions (like a video game or a car). Or he may envy something less material, like personal or physical features (such as intelligence, popularity, athletic talent, or beauty.)

Excessive and persistent envy may indicate an underlying sense of deprivation, inadequacy, unworthiness, or entitlement that comes from other sources. Your child's envy may be stimulated indirectly by an excessive interest in material belongings, modeled after family, friends, or the general culture. Or it may be indirectly stimulated by an intense attention to the social pecking order and a strong competitive outlook, both of which promote seeing individual differences in the simplistic terms of "winners" and "losers." Again, this attitude may be encouraged by family, school, or the culture in general.

Possible intervention:

- Tell your child that you are familiar with the feeling of envy.
- Express your understanding of how painful this emotion can be. This may help your child feel less alone and maybe less envious.
- Talk with your child about the links between excessive materialism, intense competition, and envy.
- If envy remains persistent, generalized, and disruptive of relationships, psychotherapy may help reduce the negative effects.

Fantasizing: Fantasizing is the use of imagination, like "daydreaming." Your child understands that the fantasy is inside her mind and does not confuse it with reality. Fantasies are a normal way to deal with distressing feelings and situations and to experience pleasure. It only is worrisome if used in the extreme: when it is so frequent that it interferes with normal childhood activities, or when the content of the fantasies is overly aggressive and sexualized.

Your child is most likely to fantasize excessively when unhappy. She may think that she can only find relief in her imagination. Feeling unable to bring about changes in the world around her, she imagines scenes or stories that bring a positive outcome to her misery. Fantasizing happens most in young children who typically have limited influence on their world. Their fantasies can be vague and all-purpose. For example, your daughter may imagine that some day she will prove to others that she is successful and that they will admire her and want to be her friend. Sometimes the fantasies are specific and are elaborately dramatized. For example, she may imagine that she hits the winning home run for her favorite baseball team, or that a boy she has a crush on will fall in love with her because of some daring act.

Sometimes fantasies show up in speech, writing, or drawings. Your child may be reacting to some very stressful or traumatic experience that has not yet resolved. For example, a 12-year-old boy's father was a traveling salesman and died suddenly. The boy asked me frequently if I had traveled to specific different cities. It turned out that he fantasized that his father was still alive and traveling from city to city. He thought that if I had gone to those cities, perhaps I might have seen his father.

Excessive fascination with horror movies or violent video games may indicate underlying troubled fantasies. Those fantasies may be a reaction to disturbing real-life experiences that have stirred up feelings of rage and helplessness. Your child may be trying to work out those difficulties through the use of fantasy.

Possible intervention: The heightened use of fantasy may be a normal stage in development, a characteristic of your child (that is, highly imaginative), or a disruption or disorder in development. Fantasizing may not be of concern unless accompanied by other worrisome symptoms.

- If your child has an active fantasy life, don't tease her or belittle her about it.

- If your child wishes to share her fantasies, listen attentively and respectfully.

- Try to encourage age-appropriate social outlets for her fantasizing, like making up plays with others, or getting involved with a creative arts group after school or at your place of worship.

- If your child's fantasies are accompanied by withdrawal from peers or an increase in angry outbursts, seek professional consultation.

- If your child's fantasies seem real to her, see **Delusions** above.

Fears: These emotionally painful states, which we all experience, are associated with feeling intensely anxious and overwhelmed in response to some specific external situations. Common fears are part of growing up: fear of the dark, of being left alone, of being unloved.

Your child may experience fears in the presence of whatever he is afraid of, for example when meeting a big dog. Or, he may imagine being frightened in the future: he may not want to go down a street because he *fears* meeting a big dog. Either way, your son basically is worried that the "dangerous" event will lead to unbearable physical or emotional pain. He also fears that he will not be able to protect himself. If your child has many fears, he likely feels that the emotional or external demands placed upon him are more than he can handle.

The feared object may be something specific and literal (a dog) or more symbolic. For example, fear of taking a bath and being sucked down the drain may represent a fear of losing control, being overwhelmed, and not sufficiently protected. The more irrational fears are the most concerning (see **Obsessions, Avoidant behavior**).

Possible intervention:

- Do not tease or make fun of a child who is having irrational fears. The fear will still persist, but the child will feel less willing to talk about it.

- Validate your child's fear—"I know that the dark in the basement seems very scary to you"—but also find ways to address the irrationally feared situation: "Let's think of ways to help you overcome your fear of the dark basement."

- If you have an irrational fear like your child's, acknowledge it. You can then work together on it rather than trying to push your child to overcome a fear that you share.

- Consider behavioral therapy to help your child develop a safe plan for confronting particularly debilitating fears.

- If the fear isn't responsive to other interventions and prevents your child from doing activities that are good for his development, that he wants to do, or that keep him from being with others, consider medication.

Fighting: If your child gets into frequent physical fights, she may have a lot of underlying anger. She may blame the fights on others.

In some cases the other person is merely a stand-in. For instance, your child may feel angry with someone in the family, but take her anger out on someone at school or in the neighborhood. Sometimes fighting is a way to cope with conflict that has been learned from family members or others. Frequent fighting may reflect the fact that your child has not developed better ways to cope with her feelings and not learned how to use language as a way to deal with conflict.

Possible intervention:

- If fighting is taking place inside and outside the home, ask yourself why your child feels so much anger.

- Language may provoke a fight but can also prevent a fight. Help your child learn to ask for help and not get pulled into others' negative behavior.

- Talk about the sources of anger (see **Anger**).

- If most of your child's fighting takes place outside the home, you may want to ask yourself what angry feelings are not being expressed in the home setting. What is the family's way of dealing with anger?

- Encourage your child to develop better conflict-resolution skills.

- Consider an anger management program through local clinics. Such programs, through direct teaching and group experience, focus on ways to cope with angry feelings, challenge ideas that maintain angry behavior, and provide opportunities to practice change.

- Persistent anger may indicate an underlying emotional disorder; if the preceding interventions seem ineffective, consult with a child mental health specialist.

Fire setting: Many children, especially boys, are interested in fire. They may be fascinated by its intensity and heat. Or they may be drawn to the qualities that are connected to fire symbolically: its spontaneity and explosiveness, power and ferocity.

Many factors contribute to fire setting, such as excessive **Impulsivity** and poor judgment, immature social and emotional development, and alienation from adult authority (see **Disobedience**). Fire setting may be the outward symptom of an underlying disorder, such as **Depression**. Or there may be a psychological connection to past physical or sexual abuse that shows up as a problem caring about others or accepting and following safety rules (see **Trauma-related symptoms**). Your child also may have an obsession with fire that he compulsively acts out.

A child who is excessively preoccupied with fire or who purposely sets a destructive fire needs immediate professional evaluation, as does a child who accidentally sets a serious fire.

Possible intervention:

- Seek an educational program for children at your local fire department.

- Make sure matches and lighters are not available in the home.

- Reward your child for returning to you any matches or lighters he finds accidentally.

- Tell your child, in a calm state, that you want to help him not set fires and you will do whatever is necessary to eliminate this dangerous behavior because you are concerned about the harm that can come to him, you, and others.

- Seek professional consultation to help identify the specific factors driving the behavior and to suggest possible treatments.

Gender identity confusion: Your child may know from an early age that he is a boy. But you may hear him say or do things that express his disappointment or discomfort with his body gender. For girls, cross-gender dressing is regarded as a normal developmental phase: they are "tomboys." But for boys, there is no similar phase.

Cross-gender dressing may be a sign of gender identity confusion, which is different from **Homosexuality**. Homosexuality is the presence of a sexual attraction to others of the same gender/sex. Gender identity confusion is disappointment or discomfort with one's birth gender.

Such a problem is not a matter of your child's choice. It is the outcome of complex causes outside of your child's awareness. In some situations of gender identity confusion, birth abnormalities of the genitals may be a major factor. Yet often the causes are not easily identified.

Gender identity confusion can cause your child great distress and trigger a psychological disorder, such as **Depression**. School peers may tease or shun your child because of behavior that expresses his gender identity confusion. This adds more stress to an already stressful situation.

Possible intervention:

- Do not let this problem dominate how you think about or interact with your child.

- Psychodynamic psychotherapy may help your child cope better with the fear, shame, and anger that are often a part of gender identity confusion.

- If you feel a great sense of guilt or responsibility for your child's problem, you may want to enter counseling to help you cope better with this difficult issue and be more helpful to your child.

- In counseling, discuss how to address the impact of this disorder on your child's social life and perhaps on your own.

- No medication addresses this primary difficulty. However, medication may help to address disorders that can result from this problem, such as **Depression**.

Hair pulling: Hair pulling, along with nail biting, is a **Compulsion** that is generally thought of as an outlet for an excess of anxiety. A child may pull out eyelashes or discrete scalp hairs. This behavior is best addressed when your child wants to stop it.

Possible intervention: This behavior frequently occurs outside of your child's awareness, so helping your child become aware of the hair pulling when it happens can be an important first step.

- Do not shame your child. Call her awareness to the behavior in a compassionate manner.

- Communicate to her that you understand that it is difficult to stop such behavior.

- Use a three-step behavioral reward system: 1. increase awareness of the behavior; 2. develop an alternative behavior for tension release; and 3. reward your daughter when she stops hair pulling and uses an alternative behavior, such as squeezing a rubber ball.

- Since hair pulling is in the "compulsive disorder" continuum, medication with selective serotonin reuptake inhibitors (SSRIs) used to treat compulsions may help.

Hallucinations: A hallucination is something heard (auditory hallucination) or seen (visual hallucination) that is incorrectly experienced as coming from outside the mind, when in fact the source is from within the mind. Such experiences may be normal for a toddler who is not yet able to distinguish fantasy from reality. But for an older child or adolescent, the presence of hallucinations usually indicates a major disturbance in important psychological skills.

The reason for hallucinations is not usually known, but sometimes it is. Ongoing hallucinations, especially visual or olfactory (smell) ones, may indicate that your child has a neurological or other type of medical disorder. Hallucinations can occur when your child has a high fever and then disappear when the fever passes. Hallucinations from drugs of abuse may occur both during their usage and on withdrawal; they usually disappear shortly after the drug wears off, but not always.

Possible intervention: A child with such difficulty distinguishing inside from outside needs professional attention.

- Seek psychiatric or general medical consultation as soon as possible.

- Request a full medical evaluation for treatable causes of hallucinations.

- Medication is the core treatment for hallucinations associated with major mental illness or caused by illicit drugs.

- Most hallucinations can be fully eliminated with proper medication, but long-term psychological and social treatment is also very useful.

- To distract your child/adolescent from his hallucinations temporarily, calmly engage him in conversation.

Homosexuality: Homosexuality is sexual interest in someone of one's own gender. It is *not* considered a psychiatric disorder or a symptom that needs treatment.

Many different factors—biological, developmental, psychological, and social—contribute to sexual interest (heterosexual and homosexual). Homosexual interests or behavior may be normal in certain phases of growing up for heterosexual boys and girls, particularly during the early phases of sexual maturing. Thus it is hard to predict a child's ultimate sexual preference based upon interests and behavior while he or she is still developing psychologically.

But we do know about the psychological distress that may be associated with homosexuality. This distress commonly comes from the sense of rejection and injured self-esteem that results from the hostility and negativity of others when your child "comes out." This emotional pain may also come when your child feels different from others who are important to him or her.

Possible intervention:

- If you are having a lot of distress about your child's sexual orientation, you may find joining a parents' support group or entering psychotherapy helpful.

- If your child is firm in his or her sexual orientation, psychotherapy to address that issue generally is *not* recommended.

- If your child feels uncertain, doubtful, or conflicted about his or her sexual orientation, he or she may benefit from therapy.

- Psychotherapy may help your child cope with the stress that comes from his or her differences with heterosexual family members or peers and with the impact of the social isolation or depression that may result from the stigma sometimes attached to homosexuality.

Hostility: Your child's constant antagonistic behavior usually reflects unresolved anger that is muted or "backed up." You may experience this underlying hostility as "bad attitude," ongoing disrespect, rudeness, or chronic disobedience. He also may express hostility by destroying property or repeatedly getting into verbal or physical fights.

Possible intervention: Your child needs to develop more effective ways to cope with anger (see **Anger**).

- Help your child develop anger management techniques.

- Address any underlying emotional factors, such as depression or mood modulation disorder.

- Seek family therapy to develop better ways to tackle existing problems between particular members that often fan the fires of children's hostility.

Hyperactivity: This is a level of activity in a child that seems greater than that of his age-matched peers. It may be due to his temperamental make-up, an ongoing state of fear or anxiety, a mood disorder (such as bipolar disorder), or some combination.

When combined with attentional difficulties (see **Inattention**) and **Impulsivity**, this behavior can interfere with many aspects of your child's development. He may have problems making and keeping friends or working up to his abilities and succeeding in school. Problems effectively coping with frustration and maintaining relationships may occur if your son uses activity as his principal way of handling distressing emotions.

Possible intervention:

- Make sure your child has lots of physical outlets during the day to discharge hyperactive energy.

- For a school-aged child, keep opportunities for over-stimulation (such as large groups or rapidly changing activities) to a minimum.

- If your child is sensitive to diet and sugar intake, provide a balanced diet with limited sweets.

- If a disorder (the attention deficit hyperactivity disorder (ADHD) symptoms of inattention, impulsivity, and hyperactivity) is present, treatment with medication, the omega-3 fatty acids docosahexaenoic acid (DHA) and eicosapentaenoic acid (EPA) (see Chapter 10) and some form of psychotherapy to help with associated social and emotional problems can be very useful.

Immaturity: Psychological and social immaturity means that your child behaves in ways that are typical of a much younger child. Such immaturity may be episodic or ongoing.

Episodic regression is normal: your child regresses to a younger stage when he is under stress that brings up anger, fear, sadness, or shame which may overwhelm your child's coping skills. For example, a pre-teen getting ready to go to overnight camp for the first time might want to be tucked into bed as he was when he was younger. He may need extra reassurance about his ability to cope with his first solo experience away from home.

Ongoing immature behavior often reflects delays in your child's emotional development. This may be most obvious when you compare him to his peers. Remember that children mature at different rates. Your child's immaturity may stand out when you compare his development with your sense of how grown up you think he ought to be. Your expectations may be unreasonably high (common for first-time parents). Or your expectations may be reasonable but your child cannot meet them. You and your child may both have a hard time accepting his immaturity and wish that he were better at dealing with complex social and emotional situations.

Possible intervention: Despite your child's ongoing immaturity, he will indeed grow up.

- Talk with your child about his seeming younger than his age. Do it in a non-judgmental manner and remember that he will indeed "grow up."

- While he is "catching up" to his chronological age, you may need to help him accept that he is not as mature as either you or he wishes.

- At times, you may think that he is "too old" to require a certain kind of attention or help, yet his behavior may tell you otherwise. Provide more parental structure, time and "buffering" for stressful situations and difficult emotions.

- Psychological and social immaturity may be encouraged unintentionally by certain kinds of family interactions. If you think this is happening, seek consultation with a family therapist.

- If your child is motivated, individual therapy can help him become more aware of the emotions that contribute to immature behavior.

Impulsivity: A child who is impulsive tends to make decisions or to take action without considering possible consequences of her behavior. Impulsivity may stem from one or more factors:

- It may be due to a delay in development because of an impairment or immaturity of her nervous system.

- It may simply reflect a temperamental style.

- It may be a response to anxiety or other difficult emotional state.

- Your child may be seeking relief through some instant gratification, using immediate action to remove or temporarily overcome feelings of distress.

Your child may have an especially hard time tolerating the emotions that go with uncertainty or indecision, which are best worked through slowly and gradually. Children's impulsivity increases when there is an increase in anxiety, anger, or guilt. Times of transition and other situations of less structure predictably increase anxiety. Over-stimulating circumstances, like shopping in a mall, may lead to an increase in impulsive behavior and decreased tolerance for waiting and thinking before acting.

For example, a 13-year-old girl who is in the primary custody of her mother after her parents' highly conflicted divorce may feel increasingly anxious about visiting with her father. For her, he has been a largely absent, somewhat intimidating, but quite beloved man. She is nervous due to the conflicting emotions of fear and love raised by seeing him. The day of the visit she may impulsively cut her own hair, steal something, or behave in a way that would interfere with the visit.

Possible intervention: Younger children are more impulsive than older children. Whatever degree of impulsivity your child has, for whatever reason, it will likely decrease with development. While you're waiting for development to take over, consider these interventions:

- Look more closely at the situations that provoke anxiety. Work with your child by helping her identify emotional states that trigger impulsive behavior.

- Professional evaluation may help clarify how much your child's impulsivity is interfering with development and what some of the stressful situations are.

- If treatment is recommended, the focus may be on ways to provide more structure and order for your child.

- If an identifiable disorder, such as ADHD, an anxiety disorder, or mood disorder, may be contributing to the impulsivity, medication may be a useful part of treatment.

Inattention: Your child's delays or disruptions in the ability to focus and attend may be obvious when you compare him to his peers. Such delays can lead to the kinds of difficulties discussed under **Hyperactivity**: he may have a hard time making and keeping friends, working up to his abilities, or succeeding in school (see also "Disruption of bodily activity" in Chapter 3.)

Problems with inattention may be accompanied by blocks in cognitive development, and progress in school may be delayed (see **Learning problems/disorders**). Emotional or social development may also be blocked. **Impulsivity** often goes along with inattention. If your child is only inattentive at school, there may be a mismatch between your child's abilities and what the school is providing.

Possible intervention:

- Your child's ability to focus and attend will improve with age and development.

- When trying to help your child with his schoolwork, find out what conditions improve his focus and attention and what conditions diminish it.

- Psychopharmacological treatment, omega-3 fatty acids (see Chapter 10) and psychotherapeutic treatment may help your child (see **Hyperactivity**).

Insomnia: Your child's difficulty falling asleep, staying asleep, or waking very early are all forms of insomnia. The type of insomnia may vary depending upon the cause. Worry and anxiety often lead to difficulty falling asleep. A problem of waking up very early in the morning may be associated with depression or attention–deficit hyperactivity disorder. Past stress or trauma that took place mainly at night may also lead to insomnia.

A high level of **Anxiety** or **Separation anxiety** may cause a child to wake up from scary dreams or feel anxious about being alone with inner fears and fantasies at bedtime. If your child is young and has difficulty distinguishing between thoughts and reality, the monsters might seem quite real indeed.

A lack of good habits of preparing for sleep (such as engaging in pre-bedtime calming routines and bedtime rituals) may also contribute to insomnia.

Possible intervention:

- Develop a regular bedtime for your child. If she is young, use a calming routine or ritual before you leave the bedroom: play music, tell a story, or do another activity that is calming and can be repeated each night without much variation.

- Give your child a temporary period of extra support to help her feel safe in her bed. For example, tell her you'll check her frequently (and do so!) or sit outside her door until she falls asleep.

- Follow this period with a gradual transition to less support.

- If your child has had major problems getting to sleep, consult with your family doctor about using an herbal medicinal or prescribed medication as a helper at the start of a new bedtime routine.

Irritability: Irritability may show up as a critical tone in your child's voice when he interacts with you or in his frequent negative reaction to your suggestions. This frequently represents a low-level state of chronic anger (see **Anger** and **Hostility**).

Jealousy: This emotion is a painful mix of desire, disappointment, shame, anger, and fear. It is usually connected to a triangular relationship: your child may feel jealous toward someone who has a particular type of relationship with a third person. Your child would herself like to have that relationship and feels deprived.

Your child may imagine that involvement with the third person is a source of great satisfaction, pleasure, and pride for the person she is jealous of. Your daughter may believe that the desirable relationship would protect her from her disappointment, shame, anger, and fear. A similar fantasy of protection may be behind **Envy**, which is related to and often occurs with jealousy. **Envy** usually is focused on particular things or traits that someone else has that the envious person wants to possess (see **Envy**).

Sibling rivalry is one of the earliest experiences of jealousy. Jealousy points toward the experience of needing, but not having, a particular kind of relationship with one or both parents. The jealous child expects the relationship with one or both parents to provide ongoing feelings of safety, comfort, affirmation and pleasure that seem unattainable otherwise.

Usually jealousy is short-lived. It is a problem if your child is excessively and persistently jealous and imagines that only one particular relationship (person) can make her happy.

Possible intervention:

- Realize that jealousy is intimately linked to coping with feelings such as shame, fear, and disappointment. This may help you respond more empathically to your child.

- If sibling rivalry does not seem outweighed by sibling love and cooperation, address this by encouraging opportunities for pleasurable interactions. Do not tolerate intense sibling rivalry as "the way it is."

- If your daughter is jealous of a particular relationship or person, help her reduce the intensity of her jealousy by acknowledging and expressing disappointment, shame, anger, and fear that exist in other areas of her life.

- Consider therapy for situations of intense jealousy that create major relationship problems.

Learning problems/disorders: If your child does not seem to be learning at the expected rate (compared to his peers or his potential), there are many possible complex causes (see Chapter 3, "School-aged children: disruptions of information processing (learning)" on page 112, and Chapter 6 under "Psychological tests" on page 163).

Possible intervention:

- Tell your child that you understand and appreciate how hard he has to work to make progress.

- Seek a comprehensive evaluation, including psycho-educational, psychological, or neuropsychological testing (see Chapter 6 for detailed information about testing).

- Ask the professional doing the evaluation how you should tell your child about it.

- Consider additional services within or outside school to remedy the situation.

- Keep in mind that other symptoms requiring intervention, such as **Compulsions, Impulsivity, Rigidity**, etc., may be present with certain types of learning disorders, particularly those called non-verbal learning disorders (NVLD).

- Actively lobby for services. Since such services can be costly, school authorities may resist acknowledging the extent of the difficulties.

- Find other parents to help and support school personnel who are seeking more resources.

Lying: Lying is driven by your child's urge to misrepresent reality, usually in order to avoid something painful. Lying may also be driven by intense shame or guilt that your child has about his behavior: he may want to avoid those feelings by distorting reality. Or your child may want to avoid an intense reaction from you. If your child is very young, he may not experience the guilt and shame as coming from within, but experience it as coming solely from you.

Your child also may lie due to an urge to get something pleasurable (e.g. cookies before meals or staying at a friend's house without supervision) that he doesn't think he can get in any other way.

It is developmentally normal for a young child to lie occasionally. But when a child persistently and frequently lies, he probably has failed to develop age-appropriate methods to manage his desires. A child who lies tends to distrust his ability to get what he wants. He may feel unable to handle disappointment. He may distrust that others will understand or respond to his needs. Lying then becomes habitual.

Possible intervention:

- Your honesty with your child is the best model for his behaving honestly.
- Wonder with your child, "Why would you, a boy who can be honest and truthful, not be so at this time?"
- Don't try to "catch" or trick your child in a lie by asking him a question to which you already know the answer.
- Consider family therapy to improve communication and work together on the problem if it seems that you are getting nowhere on your own.
- If the lying is persistent and creating significant social problems, seek consultation, especially if lying is part of a larger pattern of difficulties, such as **Disobedience**, **Fire setting**, or **Stealing**.

Manipulation: Similar to and different from **Lying**, manipulation indicates your child's need to use devious means to get something that seems beyond her reach otherwise. For example, your child may ask for a ride to the mall, saying she wants to buy her sister a birthday gift; this may be true, but her main plan is to meet a boyfriend you dislike.

Underlying your child's manipulative behavior may be a feeling of impotence and a lack of skill at getting what she wants by more straightforward means. She also may have a low tolerance for frustration at not getting what she wants and at almost any cost tries to avoid the feelings of sadness or anger.

Sometimes people use the term "manipulation" about a child because her behavior is contrary to what the adult wants, and she is simply trying to get her way in a non-devious fashion. For example, your daughter cleans up her room and completes her chores with the hope of putting you in a good mood to allow her to do something which you might disapprove of. Such behavior is not manipulative; rather it is planful and strategic.

Possible intervention:

- Help your child see that the limits you are imposing are not to deprive or punish her.

- Explain the reasons for the limits. Although your child may not agree, hearing your thinking will help her feel less impotent.

- Let her know you understand her disappointment and annoyance at not getting what she wants.

- Admire any honest and direct expression of what she wants, when appropriate, even if you turn down her request.

- If you find your anger interfering with effectively addressing this problem behavior seek consultation.

Meanness: Mean behavior is experienced as hurtful, insensitive, and lacking empathy. Often a high level of **Anger** or **Hostility** is behind such actions. The behavior of the classic bully, picking on someone smaller and considerably less powerful, is an example of "mean behavior" (see **Bullying**).

People often assume that mean behavior is intentional. But your child may not view it this way. He might feel self-protective and uncared about and thus uncaring about others' feelings. A child's mean actions often occur because of a past experience of being the object of others' humiliating, demeaning, or injurious behavior. Such treatment inside the family (by siblings or adults) can have a more lasting impact than similar treatment outside the family.

Possible intervention:

- Look for current causes of **Anger**, **Jealousy**, **Envy**, and humiliation in your child's life and try to address them.

- Talk about your child's experiences of being treated meanly by others. Help him to put his painful experience into words. This can decrease the likelihood of his acting out his anger and diminish his impulse to play out his *own* past experience of being the target of mean behavior by being mean to *another* child.

- If your child seems detached and uncaring about his behavior, seek consultation.

- Consider psychotherapy to help your child with past and current feelings of being uncared for or neglected, which may underlie mean behavior.

Mood swings: The stable emotional states we call moods also have a natural change-ableness. Your child may go through predictable periods of different moods: upbeat or energetic, subdued or quiet, and balanced.

Under normal circumstances, the changes from one mood state to another are neither extreme nor rapid. However, children, particularly adolescents, sometimes go through periods of more rapid mood changes. This can be due to growth-related hormonal spurts, other physical causes, or psychological and social changes.

Normally, those times of wider or more rapid mood swings are rather infrequent and last no more than a couple of weeks.

However, your child's moods may alternate between phases of great elation or irritability and phases of depression and despair. The swing may occur slowly or quickly. Your child's behavior and functioning at either end of this mood range can cause many problems. Her moods may severely disrupt her good judgment and keep her from being able to delay her impulses and reflect on a situation. As a result, her mood swings may interfere with her ability to keep herself safe. If such extreme moods are present, she may be diagnosed with a major disorder of mood modulation, commonly referred to as *bipolar disorder*.

Often a child's quality of mood changes is an outcome of several factors which may be hard to disentangle. Do your daughter's mood swings grow largely out of situational stress? Such stress may be acute or chronic. It may be visible or hidden (such as unidentified sexual abuse). Or do the mood swings grow out of a basic problem with mood regulation connected to temperamental and developmental causes?

Possible intervention:

- Find out whether your daughter realizes that she has been having mood swings.

- If you both agree that she is having mood swings, work together to find out if there are identifiable triggers. These might be incidents like a recent stress within or outside the family, or a recent disruption in sleep routine or other bodily/physical changes.

- Address any identified causes.

- If you disagree about whether she is having mood swings, accept that your perspectives differ.

- Try to find agreement on how you will work at bridging the gap between the two viewpoints. For example, you could each keep a journal of behaviors and mood changes for a couple of weeks or a month and then compare notes.

- The discussion about symptom frequency, intensity, and consequences in Chapter 1 provides guidance about when to seek professional consultation.

- If you do consult a professional who recommends medication, read the discussion on psychopharmacological treatment in Chapter 9.

Nail biting: This compulsive behavior, along with hair pulling, is generally a way to relieve excess **Anxiety**. Nail biting is best addressed when your child wants to stop.

Possible intervention: Many interventions for hair pulling apply to nail biting:

- Do not shame your daughter. Help her become aware of the behavior in a compassionate and understanding manner.

- Tell her that you understand it is difficult to stop such behavior.

- Use a three-step behavioral reward system: 1. increase awareness of the behavior happening; 2. develop an alternative behavior for tension release; and 3. reward your daughter when she stops nail biting and instead uses an alternative behavior (such as chewing gum or some alternative activity with the hands, like drumming).

- Since nail biting might be included in the "compulsive disorder" category, medication (SSRIs) used to treat compulsions may help.

- Only paint your child's nails with a distasteful over-the-counter substance if she wants to try that method of disrupting an automatic behavior.

Nightmares: An occasional nightmare is normal and often associated with some unusual emotional stress from the day (like a horror movie that your son thought was "fun").

Frequent nightmares, however, should not be ignored. They may be part of an anxiety disorder, associated with post-traumatic stress disorder, or one symptom of a sleep pattern disorder, such as **Night terrors**.

Possible intervention:

- Find ways to increase your child's sense of night-time safety. Use calming bedtime routines, a night light, open doors, and comforting objects in bed.

- For persistent ongoing nightmares, seek professional consultation to help you identify sources of stress and deal with them (see **Sleep problems**).

Night terrors: Night terrors are present when your child wakes during the night in a state of severe fright, often with eyes wide open, screaming or thrashing about, but does not remember the event the next day.

Night terrors are more likely to occur when a child is overly tired. They usually occur about the same time each night, often shortly after your child falls asleep. By contrast, simple nightmares are often remembered the next day and happen at various times throughout the night.

Night terrors are due to a disruption of the brain's normal sleep cycle and not primarily to emotional factors. They are often time-limited.

Possible intervention:

- Change your child's bedtime to disrupt night terrors if a cycle has developed.

- If night terrors persist, your child may benefit from a brief use of medication prescribed by your pediatrician.

Obsessions: Obsessions are repetitive patterns of thinking, often with a focus on a particular topic. For example, your son may spend large parts of the day thinking about something that happened many years ago or preoccupied with worry that he will be contaminated by germs. He may say that this pattern of thinking keeps him from focusing on other things or distracts him.

Obsessive thoughts may be accompanied by any emotion: sadness or shame (as in the preoccupation with the past) or fear or terror (as in the example about contamination). Obsessive thoughts about pornographic material may be pleasurable, but often can be accompanied by intense shame and guilt.

Sometimes children perform an action to control obsessive thoughts (**Compulsions**). Compulsions may also be a magical attempt to ward off events or feelings your child finds overwhelming and dangerous. When both obsessions and compulsions are present, professionals use the term "obsessive–compulsive disorder."

From a biological perspective, obsessions are thought of as "stuck brain patterns" best treated with medication. From a psychological perspective, obsessive thoughts are seen as an off-shoot of your child's struggle to cope with difficult emotions. Fear, anger, and guilt may arise normally in one area of his life, and he may deal with them indirectly, or symbolically, in another area.

For example, he may have an obsessive thought that he has germ-contaminated hands that will endanger his family. He may have this idea while trying to cope with angry feelings towards family members whom he loves. The feelings seem very dangerous and hard to manage. His mind substitutes germs for the dangerous thoughts and feelings and he then focuses his attention on controlling the germs. His focus on the germs is an involuntary attempt to cope with his anger. He might then get stuck distractedly in this pattern instead of dealing with those feelings more directly.

Possible intervention:

- Try not to get caught up in the behavior; help your son think about what emotions are troubling him.

- If the obsessions are mild, try to identify what situation might be causing distressing emotions.

- Consider family therapy to address interpersonal sources of conflict and help everyone cope better with the symptoms.

- Seek therapy for your son to help him learn to cope with his obsessions and learn more about his emotional experience.

- Obsessions can be treated with cognitive behavioral methods; they can be somewhat more challenging than compulsive behavior.

- For more intense obsessions, consider medication to bring your child relief and to help therapy be most effective.

Oppositional behavior: Oppositional behavior is disobedient, negative, or contrary and well beyond the ordinary self-assertiveness of children or adolescents. This behavior may be characterized by a relentless challenge to others' opinions, in particular the views of authority figures.

Oppositional children are not open to the easy flow of compromise that one expects in most human relations. Instead, such a child may act as though ordinary simple requests or directions are an affront. Daily life with the child is exhausting, and a parent may often feel perplexed and worn down.

Oppositional behavior may be the result of some other untreated problem (see **Inattention**, **Hyperactivity**, **Depression**, and **Anxiety**). A child may learn oppositional behavior from a family environment of chronic arguing and conflict. In such a setting, a child may not feel that her needs are met or that she is understood.

Possible intervention:

- Usually, a pattern of oppositional behavior needs to be addressed through psychotherapy.
- Consider family therapy to tackle problems in communication and mutual understanding.
- Consider group therapy, which may help your daughter develop social skills and a tolerance for frustration/distress.
- Have your child evaluated for untreated depression, a disorder of attention, or other problems.

Pressured speech: If your child speaks very rapidly, jumping from one idea to another quickly and hardly waiting for a response, she shows "pressured speech." While most brief episodes of pressured speech indicate excitement or a high level of anxiety, such behavior that is ongoing may indicate chronic **Anxiety**, a mood disorder, or a **Hyperactivity** disorder.

Possible intervention:

- Increase your child's awareness of the pressured speech in a non-critical manner by commenting that she speaks so fast it is hard to follow.
- If the main problem is **Anxiety**, **Mood swings**, or **Hyperactivity**, see each heading in this chapter for steps you can take.
- If the episodes are prolonged and not responding to your interventions, seek professional intervention.
- If the symptom is accompanied by difficulty sleeping, poor judgments, and other disruptions in routine functioning, also seek professional intervention.

Rigidity: A child who has developed a certain way of dealing with people and situations, and finds it hard to do things in a new or different way, shows rigidity. She may resist new experiences, or find it hard to transition from one situation to another. She may experience change as threatening, or worry about "falling apart" if she does not keep the rigid pattern.

A tendency toward rigidity may be a temperamental trait, perhaps connected to underlying **Shyness**. Or your child may have developed rigidity as a coping style when she felt overwhelmed by change and new information. If your child has a significant learning disorder or problems coping with social interactions because of a difficulty reading social cues, she may appear rigid. A sudden or marked increase in your child's level of rigidity may indicate an increase in **Anxiety**, the development of an underlying **Depression**, or an intensification of **Compulsions** that are part of an obsessive–compulsive disorder. A child with an intense persistent pattern of rigidity that is accompanied by language, motor, and social problems may receive a diagnosis of pervasive developmental disorder or autism.

A high level of rigidity can cause frequent confrontations with authority figures who want some change in routine from your child. She may view the change as unwanted and as too dramatic or sudden. Rigidity may lead to a pattern of **Oppositional** or **Avoidant behavior**.

Possible intervention: Rigidity can wear on all family members, including your child. The better your child's self-esteem, the less likely she is to exhibit rigidity.

- Understand that her rigidity comes from a need to protect herself. This may help you find some compassion and move beyond your own rigid stance.

- Help your child cope by sensitively showing her a sense of humor when fitting.

- Do not shame your child about her rigidity.

- Leave extra time to work through a situation with your child, so that you are not feeling pressured yourself.

- Consider family therapy. Usually, coping patterns are influenced by interactions within the family; therapy may help all family members work together better by finding strategies for dealing with conflict that respects all styles within the family.

- Consider professional treatment directed at an underlying **Depression**, **Anxiety** disorder (such as social phobia) or obsessive–compulsive disorder.

Rudeness: Rudeness is insensitivity to the wishes and feelings of others. This may reflect a high level of self-centeredness, a sudden or chronic angry state, or poor social skills (see **Hostility**). Your child may have poor social skills due to poor social training or some impairment that keeps your child from grasping (intellectually or emotionally) the rules of proper social relations. Such insensitivity may be present in children who are going through a prolonged stressful transition, experiencing a delay in development, or coping with a major mental disorder.

Possible intervention:

- Do not shame your child about his rudeness.
- Comment in a non-judgmental way that he needs to be more sensitive to the feelings of others and offer alternative ways for him to express himself in such a situation.

Frank was a developmentally delayed child who frequently greeted others with some rude name-calling. Usually the greeting exaggerated their physical appearance: "Hi fatty," or "Hi baldy." His father told him in a matter of fact way that such descriptive comments were hurtful and that he only needed to greet others by saying "Hi" or "Hello."

- Seek professional assistance to help your child identify and address the underlying emotions and thoughts contributing to this rudeness.

Running away: Many young children may express their hurt and anger with a parent by talking about, planning, or actually running away. Teenagers who run away are expressing similar hurt and anger. Either they have not developed adequate skills for communicating their misery or they experience their home environment as intolerably toxic. Running away is a form of communication and an attempt at problem-solving.

Possible intervention:

- Respond in an empathic way to your child's distress when she talks about or returns from running away.
- Do not belittle or shame your child.
- Realize that running away is her way to express her hurt and anger.
- Do not respond with restrictions or consequences alone, since these likely will increase your child's sense of alienation.
- In a caring manner, communicate your worry about her safety.
- If running away recurs, seek consultation to help you and your child determine the source of the anger and distress and find effective ways to address it.

- Particularly with adolescents, do not let this behavior become a pattern; seek help sooner rather than later.

School avoidance: Your child may experience, imagine, or invent reasons not to go to school: medical and physical complaints, or exaggerated stories about the dangers he faces at school. If the dangers your child describes seem plausible, you may be drawn into elaborate measures aimed at protecting your child.

School avoidance usually is an expression of **Separation anxiety**: your child may fear going to school in a large part because he fears not being at home or with family where he feels safest. He may be unaware of the source of his fear or may be too confused or embarrassed to express it.

School avoidance may also indicate that your child has an undiagnosed learning disorder. He may feel ashamed and anxious because he isn't learning as others do and has no way to cope with this.

Possible intervention:

- Firmly support school attendance. Just as you would go to work if you were in minor physical discomfort, you can reasonably expect your child to go to school.

- Provide clear definitions of when and why your child may stay home from school. For example, if he often complains of vague illness, tell him that he can stay home if he has a fever, but not if his temperature is normal.

- Communicate clearly so school staff understand that your child's difficulty comes from anxiety, not simple opposition. Then everyone involved can support and encourage your anxious child.

- Ask yourself whether family stresses that have not been openly identified may be a factor. Your child may be responding to family issues but not talking about them. For example, your son may feel excluded following the birth of a sibling who gets to stay home with mother. Or he may be responding to conflict at home and wonder if everyone is safe when he is away.

- Consider family therapy to address your child's fears about separation.

- When symptoms are particularly intense and long-lasting, medication may help to lower your child's anxiety level or eliminate panic attacks associated with **Separation anxiety**.

School behavior problems: These may be due to trouble in one or more school areas: academic work, peer interactions, or authority relationships. Problems in one area can influence any of the other two areas. Almost any significant difficulty in the area of mood, anxiety, activity level, or attention can also lead to school behavior problems.

Possible intervention:

- Consult with school authorities early.

- Consider assessment, including evaluation by a specialist outside the school, to help you and your child understand the underlying problems. For example, your child may have a non-verbal (meaning more perceptual or visua–spatial, rather than language-based) type learning disorder (see Chapter 3, "School-aged children: disruption of information processing (learning)" on page 112, and Chapter 6, "Psychological tests" on page 163).

- Pay extra attention to behavioral problems that show up only at school and not at home. Such a situation does not automatically mean that the problem resides primarily at school. Your child may be hiding problems from you and acting out home-related difficulties in the public arena.

Self-injury/self-abuse: A younger child may injure herself by running into walls, banging her head, or picking at scabs. An adolescent may cut, burn, or otherwise hurt herself. Such behaviors are purposeful, yet also have an involuntary and driven quality. In younger children, feelings connected to the experience of neglect and deprivation often underlie such behavior. In teens, such behavior may indicate that your child feels overwhelmed with self-punitive thoughts and emotions.

The act of self-injury may be a physical way to get relief from what feels like an overwhelming state of emotional pain and agitation. The emotional pain is usually a jumble of terror, anger, humiliation, guilt, and grief.

Paradoxically, self-injury may also be a way to get relief from numbness, which may be a feeling of deadness and insensitivity to any feelings whatsoever. Numbness can arise as an involuntary and self-protective response to repeated episodes of tor- turous emotions.

Possible intervention:

- Avoid adding to your child's pain; do not respond punitively.

- Respond to the communication about her deeper emotional distress by seeking professional help QUICKLY.

Separation anxiety: Separation anxiety may show up as **School avoidance** or diffi- culty having sleep-overs at friends' houses. Inborn temperament (see **Shyness**) may be a factor. A parent's own anxiety about separating from the child may trigger sepa- ration anxiety in the child. And some children just take longer to develop the sense of confidence, self-reliance, and trust required to be away from "protectors."

Possible intervention:

- Offer your child extra time, recognition, support, and encouragement for his difficulty at being on his own.

- If separation anxiety causes your child major distress or keeps him from doing things he needs to do despite your support, seek professional consultation.

- Psychotherapy can help you and your child understand some of the causes of your child's vulnerability to separation and deal with them.

- Consider psychodynamic psychotherapy and cognitive behavioral therapy (CBT). CBT techniques provide focused interventions that are very useful for diminishing separation anxiety.

- If your child is stuck in immobilizing anxiety or subject to states of panic and rage that come up during separations, medication may be necessary (see also **Anxiety**.)

Sexual preoccupation: Sexual preoccupation is caused by a child's anxiety about his own sexual identity (see **Gender identity confusion** and **Homosexuality**) or worries about sexual contact with others. Your child may frequently ask questions, show high interest in pornographic material, or write and draw pictures of a sexual nature.

A strong interest in sexual matters may indicate normal development, a variation of normal development, or a disorder. The meaning varies depending upon your child's age and on the nature and intensity of the preoccupation.

In a young child, such preoccupation is of major concern and suggests that your child may have experienced inappropriate over-stimulation and exposure to sexual material (through television, video, movies, and audio recordings, or as a result of a traumatic sexual encounter). Sudden dramatic changes in your child's behavior may be due to the intense fear, helplessness, and disorganization that commonly follow sexual trauma. A normally communicative child may keep a traumatic experience a secret out of fear, shame, guilt, and confusion. If a traumatic sexual encounter has occurred, your child may also have had inappropriate sexual behavior with others.

In adolescents, sexual preoccupation may be normal, and usually does not come to parents' attention dramatically. If it does come to parents' attention, it may be because your adolescent is having a particularly hard time coping with sexual feelings and gender differences. Of course, a sexually traumatic experience may also be an issue, and all that was said earlier about sudden changes in behavior or communication in a child who experiences sexual trauma applies to an adolescent too. A total absence of sexual interest may also indicate any of the preceding kinds of difficulties.

Sexual preoccupation may be related to other treatable conditions, such as obsessive–compulsive disorder, depression, or excessive mood swings.

Possible intervention:

- Shelter your younger child from over-stimulation and exposure to inappropriate sexual material through television, videos, movies, and audio recordings. Talk with your older child/adolescent who is exposed to this material about his views on this matter and share your views.

- If you have ill-defined concerns about the intensity or nature of your child's sexual interests, seek consultation to clarify your concerns.

- If your child's sexual preoccupation seems out of the norm and is part of other emotional and behavioral troubles, seek ongoing treatment.

- If your child's sexual preoccupations lead him to behave sexually inappropriately, seek professional consultation immediately.

- If you suspect sexual trauma of your child, also seek professional consultation immediately.

- In the absence of inappropriate behavior or specific symptoms of concern, be even more tactful than usual with your adolescent child when raising your concerns and talking about this personal arena.

Shame: Shame is a normal emotion that can become overdeveloped and come up frequently or intensely. Intense shame may contribute to excessive withdrawal, avoidance, and oppositional behavior. Many anxiety states involve the fear of being shamed or, its twin, not being "perfect."

Shame may lead to seemingly paradoxical kinds of action, such as showing off excessively or being antisocial. Your child may act like he doesn't care what others think as a way of coping with the fear of again feeling the shame that comes with social rejection. Shame is often accompanied by anger; this is why so many adolescents become furious at being "dissed" (disrespected).

Possible intervention:

- Don't tease your child who already feels shame. This will only lead to further shame and can trigger an angry response.

- Kindness and understanding are usually the most helpful immediate responses to shame.

- Foster your child's confidence and self-esteem. Help him develop his natural skills and interests so he has areas of personal competence. When he experiences a sense of self-worth and appropriate pride, his tendency to feel shame is diminished.

Showing off: Many children display some degree of showing off and seeking excessive attention. This is particularly so for young children whose ability to maintain a positive balance in self-esteem is fragile and dependent upon positive acknowledgment from others. A tendency to show off may be part of your child's temperament; it is common in a child with an exuberant and dramatic/outgoing nature.

Your child also may seek excessive attention when feeling lonely, fearful of being socially rejected, or underappreciated. Inflated feelings of importance may be a defense against feeling inadequate. If your child tends to show off, he may have a history of feeling either much overvalued or much undervalued in his family. Whatever the reasons, your child may behave like he needs more than a usual amount of positive attention from others.

Showing off may be due to an unusually elevated mood. If such a mood is chronic, your child may have a mood disorder: rapid and strong **Mood swings** from feelings of depression and inadequacy to feelings of excitement and inflated importance.

Possible intervention:

- Figure out whether the behavior is a stage in development or a sign of some problem needing more attention. If it is a developmental stage, the behavior has a less intense quality to it and it diminishes when you give your child more support and nurturing. If showing off is linked to a problematic pattern, your child's behavior seems more driven and will not respond as well to simple interventions.

- Don't shame your child as a way of curbing the behavior. Comment non-judgmentally, "It seems right now that you'd like some extra time and attention."

- Seek consultation if there are other symptoms of concern or if the showing off causes major problems with peers or in school.

Shyness: This personality characteristic seems to be due primarily to a child's inborn temperament. However, like all inborn traits, it is influenced by, and influences, a child's social experiences. It may be associated with a high level of **Anxiety** and may contribute to social withdrawal.

Possible intervention:

- Respect your child's temperamental style, while at the same time supporting her being with others rather than withdrawing.

- If this condition interferes with your child making and keeping friends, consider consultation for psychotherapy.

- Consider medication for **Anxiety**, which may accompany intense shyness and which may show up as avoidance of social contact (see **Separation anxiety**.)

Sleep problems: There are five common causes to your child's difficulty falling asleep. First, it may be related to anxiety about being alone. This anxiety may be a problem just in the evening, not during the day. Second, your child may not have developed good patterns for settling into sleep. Third, she may fear being asleep. Since sleep is a time of diminished control, a child who likes a lot of control may become very anxious before entering into a sleep state when she has less control. Fourth, your child may have a history of nightmares that makes her anxious about going to sleep. Finally, sleep problems may be caused by a generalized high level of **Anxiety**, a **depressed** mood or a past experience of some acute stress or trauma that happened at night or bedtime (see Chapter 3, "Disruption of bodily routine").

Possible intervention:

- Develop a regular bedtime for your child and stick with it.

- If your child is young, use a calming routine or ritual before you leave the bedroom. This might include reading quietly together, listening to relaxing music (a music box for example), or quietly talking to your child with the bedroom lights out.

- Do not let your child watch TV or play at the computer for 15–30 minutes before bed.

- Give your child extra support. For example, sit in the darkened room or just outside the door until your child falls asleep. For late night problems, walk your child back to bed rather than having him go back alone.

- Once your child has a sense of safety, gradually transition to less support.

- Medication to induce sleepiness (see Chapter 9) may decrease anxiety around sleep and let your child begin to develop a routine more easily.

- Address the symptoms of excessive fear or depression through personal interventions (see **Fears** and **Depression** above) or by seeking psychotherapy for your child.

Soiling: Soiling—when your child defecates in his underwear beyond the usual age of toilet training—has more than one cause. One common factor is immature development. Children with this factor often seem younger than their age. If this is a factor for your child, he might seem awkward in his gross and fine muscle movements, as well as awkward socially. He might frequently cope with his emotions like a younger child and have difficulty managing strong emotions, especially fear and anger.

Another factor is a failure to develop good bowel hygiene (regular bowel movements), which in turn may contribute to chronic constipation. Then, because of the constipation, stool leaks around the blockage and produces soiling.

A third factor is a psychological stress at the very time that bowel training is taking place (such as the birth of a younger sibling or a parent's prolonged absence). The emotional upset may interfere with the development of good bowel control.

Whatever the factors, soiling is present when your child simply and unselfconsciously has a bowel movement in his pants, or does not use the toilet when necessary and has overflow in his underclothes. Most commonly, your child will hide the soiled underclothes under the bed, in the closet, etc.

You may unintentionally find yourself in an emotionally charged control battle with your son. What may start out as your *response* to the soiling can become a *contributory cause* to the soiling. This can promote conflict and oppositional behavior in other spheres of your child's life (see Chapter 3, "Disruption of bodily routine").

Possible intervention:

- Consult with your pediatrician or family practitioner, who will decide whether or not further medical testing is needed to discover medical causes of this problem.

- Help your child develop good bowel hygiene. Have a regular toilet time (usually after meals) and make sure that his daily diet has plenty of roughage and fluids.

- Encourage your child to sit on the toilet at regular times each day. Reward his cooperation. Children with soiling problems often become "toilet phobic" and can resist sitting on the toilet.

- Ask your child's medical doctor about stool softeners, which may help while your child is developing regular toileting habits.

- Consider psychotherapy to help your child deal with the psychological or emotional causes of soiling.

- Consider parent counseling or psychotherapy if you find yourself getting into a "battle of wills" around this issue.

Stealing: A young child who takes something that is not hers may not understand property ownership clearly. Or she may just have difficulty containing her desire of the moment. This is more often due to immaturity than to a problem with moral development.

An older child who steals may feel deprived and entitled to take whatever she wants. Repeated stealing may be part of a particular style that your child developed to deal with feeling worthless, insignificant, or wicked. Instead of talking about such feelings, she impulsively or deliberately acts them out. This pattern may evolve from an inability to use adults or peers to help with such feelings.

A repeated pattern of stealing also may signal an emotional problem, such as **Depression** or **Mood swings**, or a problem with **Impulsivity**.

Possible intervention:

- As with lying, wonder with your child, "Why would you, a girl who can be honest and understands that stealing is wrong, not be honest at this time?"
- Provide natural consequences, such as having your child return or replace what was stolen and make amends to the person stolen from.
- If stealing is part of a larger pattern of difficulties, such as **Disobedience**, **Fire setting**, or **Lying**, seek professional consultation.

Suicidality: This type of behavior, including verbal threats or self-injurious actions, is *both* communication (the proverbial "cry for help") *and* an expression of inner distress. Your child may be overwhelmed, unable to communicate the depth of the despair, and feel terribly alone. He may feel depressed, hopeless, stuck, and unloved. He may not know how to communicate his suffering and need for help appropriately. It is not true that those who talk about suicide never seriously attempt it.

Suicidality is a characteristic symptom of **Depression**; it may also be present with other disorders that can be accompanied by feelings of hopelessness and despair, such as chronic **Anxiety** or panic disorder.

Possible intervention:

- Always take suicidal words and actions seriously.
- Remember that your child is usually suffering a lot if he is at the point of feeling suicidal.
- Do not dismiss the "cry for help," even if it seems manipulative and exaggerated.
- Always seek professional intervention or consultation.

Tantrums: Tantrums are a display of anger that usually reflect overwhelming inner misery with fear, shame, and disappointment. Before the tantrum, your child probably feels isolated and like no one understands her. Having no better way to communicate this distress and ask for help, she erupts into a tantrum.

Your child may have a low frustration tolerance due to **Immaturity** and a failure to develop the skills for communicating distress.

Possible intervention:

- Strengthen the positive elements in your relationship with your child and improve your understanding of what overwhelms her.
- Wait until the tantrum has passed. Then tenderly go over the specific triggers of the event with your child. If you and your child better understand what led to the tantrum, you may be able to find better ways

for both of you to deal with such situations. This works better with an older child capable of "cause and effect" thinking.

- Even if the tantrum seems manipulative, focus more on the distress that provoked it.

- Use "time out" to give your child an opportunity to settle down, pull herself together, and think about what happened (rather than as a punishment).

- Seek consultation if tantrums go on for a long time (an hour or more), occur frequently (many times a day) over a long period of time (weeks), or are unresponsive to ordinary interventions.

Trauma-related symptoms: Any situation can be traumatic if it evokes a state of terror and helplessness and is associated with the thought that there is a threat of death, serious bodily injury, or abandonment. Even if you "realistically" see the event as not so threatening, your child may view the situation differently. Your child's internal, involuntary reaction is what primarily determines whether or not trauma-related symptoms develop.

Life-threatening accidents, physical and sexual abuse, or exposure to violent events and painful medical procedures may result in trauma-related symptoms. Surgical procedures, especially complicated ones that may be repeated, are more often traumatic for young children than adults realize.

Symptoms following a traumatic experience may be acute and relatively short-lived, long-term, or delayed. Symptoms may show up as a hyper-alert, vigilant, and over-stimulated state, a constricted, numb, and withdrawn state, or as an alternation between those two states. Your child may experience nightmares and sudden disturbing images (flashbacks) that recreate the experience of the traumatic incident. She may also have exaggerated emotions, sudden startling, abrupt mood swings, and temper **Tantrums** or rage reactions.

Trauma may cause a range of long-term complex symptoms that interfere with normal development. For example, trauma may lead to an **Eating disorder** (a disruption in the task of managing the body) or problems with sustaining friendships (a disruption in the task of managing relationships). It also may result in ongoing rapid **Mood swings** or rage attacks (a disruption in balancing emotions) or in frequent "spacing out" (a disruption in processing information).

Possible intervention:

- Seek professional consultation quickly if trauma-related symptoms are present or if you know that your child has experienced an event that could evoke the above symptoms.

- If your child is undergoing surgery, consider psychological consultation for you and your child, before and after the procedure, to reduce the chances that the event will be traumatic.

- If you have a history of sexual or physical abuse in your past and have not had treatment, seek therapy. Children whose parents have been abused are at an increased risk for similar experiences.

Tics: These repetitive, involuntary, brief small muscle movements generally do not have psychological origins, but may be intensified by **Anxiety**. Motor tics tend to involve the upper body, neck, and head. They may be accompanied by vocal tics such as repeated coughing or clearing of the throat.

Tourette's syndrome is a collection of symptoms that includes motor and vocal tics. The vocal tics can be quite complex and may include repetitive words or phrases. Tics may lead to psychological symptoms like **Shame** or **Avoidance**.

Possible interention:

- If the tics are at a low level, do not bring much attention to them.

- Low frequency tics, if not creating difficulties, generally do not require medication.

- Consider medication for the more severe and disruptive tics that can be part of Tourette's syndrome.

- If you are more distressed by this symptom than your child is, consult a professional to help you manage your feelings about your child's symptom.

Wetting: Night-time wetting (bedwetting/enuresis) is usually a matter of maturity: it takes time for a child to grow into night-time bladder control. This rate of maturing is probably inherited; thus a parent of a bedwetter also often has a history of childhood bedwetting.

Daytime wetting, like **Soiling**, may be due to one of the following: immature development and a failure to register bladder sensations; difficulty with attention; and difficulty managing strong emotions like anxiety.

Usually, bedwetting is not caused by psychological problems, but is thought of as a delay in development, which means that your child will outgrow it. However, bedwetting may lead to psychological symptoms such as shame, avoidance of sleepovers with peers, and a feeling of inadequacy. Bedwetting can be very trying for all involved and lead to conflict with adults, which in turn can lead to an increase in bedwetting (see Chapter 3, "Disruption of bodily routine").

Possible intervention:

- Consider medication to help your child with night-time or daytime wetting if he is at least five or six years old. Before then, wetting is considered normal.

- Consider using a behavioral tool, such as an alarm that rings when the mattress gets wet. Your child must really want to stop bedwetting for the alarm method to succeed. He may resist using it properly because he is uncomfortable waking up in the middle of the night.

- If conflict with adults results, seek family therapy to iron out the differences and get everyone on the same side (see Chapter 8).

Whining: Although your child is very dependent on you, he also has his own desires. When his desires are not met, he can feel caught between two opposing emotional reactions. On the one hand, he experiences disappointment and anger with you for not meeting his needs. On the other hand, he loves you and fears your anger if he expresses *his* anger. Whining represents a muted expression of this emotional mix. While whining is more annoying than worrisome, it may indicate that your child is having a hard time coping with his emotions.

With development and maturity, your child will become more able to meet his own needs, more able to communicate his desires to others, and will develop better frustration tolerance. With these changes, he will probably stop whining.

Possible intervention:

- Let your child know that you understand his dilemma.

- Further your child's emotional independence by encouraging him to openly, but respectfully, express his opinion or view that differs from yours.

- Encourage him to take acceptable steps to meet his own needs.

- Help your child improve his communication skills.

- Provide extra support and clear limits.

- While whining can be quite annoying, do not seek consultation unless you cannot contain your anger and it interferes with good parenting, or the whining is accompanied by some other worrisome symptom.

Withdrawal: Pulling back or away may be the reaction of a basically shy child dealing with social or psychological stress. This response is often seen with **Avoidant behavior** or **Depression**. In a small percentage of adolescents, withdrawal may indicate a major psychiatric disorder, especially if accompanied by poor hygiene. Extreme withdrawal and avoidance may be due to recent sexual or physical trauma.

Withdrawal and avoidance may go unrecognized as problems because the suffering behind these behaviors is not easily experienced by others. This contrasts with angry and aggressive behavior that more clearly communicates a feeling of misery.

Possible intervention: Even if your child's withdrawal has been a response style for much of her life, each and every episode of withdrawal is a response to something specific. The particular situation from which she withdraws probably triggers feelings of being overwhelmed, unsafe, or at the very least, very uncomfortable.

- Try to understand her experience. Ask about her feelings and thoughts concerning a specific incident of withdrawal. This will help you understand her more than if you think of the behavior as "just her way."

- Help your daughter find more skillful ways to deal with her distress, such as learning to use her words to communicate about it, or using a journal to provide a safe place to express and reflect upon her feelings.

- If your daughter's withdrawal seems to have come on suddenly, it may be associated with some significant emotional upheaval. Talk with her about her experience.

- If you suspect depression, trauma, or some other emotional problem, seek consultation to address her distress.

Worries: see **Fears** and **Anxiety**

* * *

In this chapter, the discussion of a specific "red flag" sometimes included a brief statement or two about the symptom from a developmental perspective. The next chapter will help you think more deeply from a developmental viewpoint: that is, how the symptom may come from a delay, disruption, or distortion of a normal task in growing up.

Chapter 3

DISRUPTIONS IN DEVELOPMENT: THE WHOLE CHILD

The previous chapter focused on specific symptoms or "red flags" but did not usually take into account your child's age or link the symptom to a normal developmental task. In this chapter, I help you think about your child's symptom from a developmental viewpoint: how the symptom comes from a delay, disruption, or distortion of a normal task in growing up.

There is a lot more to your child than his problem behaviors or feelings. The problem areas and all the rest of your child make up your "whole child," the person who is trying to grow up, learn how best to adapt to the world, and get his individual needs met. Holding on to this larger "whole child" developmental view, while also being alert to the disruptions and problems, will let you take better steps towards helping your child with whatever difficulty is present. One of the hardest parts of parenting is figuring out what in your child is disruption and needs intervention and what is a normal part of development and will largely change on its own over time. I hope that this chapter will help you do just that.

Throughout this chapter I use the term "disruption" rather than the term "disorder." Typically, the term "disorder" is used when many specific symptoms occur together. For example, a "depressive disorder" involves emotional symptoms (such as prolonged sadness) and physical symptoms (such as trouble with sleeping or eating). The short-hand term for "depressive disorder" is simply "depression."

I prefer to use the term "disruption," because it brings your attention to the arena of function as well as to the symptom of dysfunction. A child's "job" in growing up is to become competent in managing the body, emotions, relationships, and information processing. I consider problems with smooth functioning in those areas a "disruption."

Organization of Chapter 3

The first part of this chapter is a discussion of the developmental perspective: its importance and the benefits derived from it. The remaining material in this chapter—symptoms from a developmental perspective—is arranged in two ways. The first is by age: toddler, preschool, school-aged, and adolescent. Your child is constantly changing: physically, emotionally, and intellectually. Generally, a child's age gives us a rough idea of what changes have happened (development) and what is yet to come.

The second way is by the tasks involved in growing up: managing the body, emotions, relationships, and processing information about the world. If your child has problems in more than one area, they are likely connected, even though the intensity or seriousness of the difficulties may vary from area to area.

Thus, each age grouping is divided into the four basic task areas. For each area, I first describe the major normal task, highlighted by the use of *italics*. Then I discuss some common problems. For example, I first describe a developmental task for a school-aged child in the area of engaging in relationships and then discuss some problems in that area.

For each area I address a few of the more common disruptions/symptoms. The examples will help you view your child's difficulties in a new and useful way and learn a fresh approach for thinking about other symptoms as well.

The importance of a developmental perspective

It is helpful to look at any symptom in a child from a developmental perspective, even a symptom that may have strong biological or genetic causes. This helps a parent keep three important questions in mind:

1. What is my child trying to accomplish or having to cope with?
2. What does the symptom have to do with my child's particular stage of development?
3. What does my child need in order to move successfully beyond this particular problem?

These questions will help you see the difficulty from your child's point of view. This has two benefits. First, your child is less likely to feel alone, frightened, or strange because of the problem or symptom. Second, if you more easily understand your child's experience, you are more likely to bring your adult knowledge to where your child needs it most.

There are other benefits to a developmental perspective. By asking what a specific symptom means for a child of a particular age, it becomes easier to distinguish what is within the normal range and what is problematic. It also helps you remember that your child is always working at many different tasks or "jobs" that are part of each stage of growing up. These countless tasks fall into four main categories:

1. managing the body and adjusting to its changing nature
2. dealing with compelling emotions and thoughts
3. engaging in relationships
4. learning about and coping with the outside world.

At times, these tasks can give your child great joy and help her feel confident. At other times, these tasks are simply part of the hard work of growing up.

Is your child primarily having difficulty *managing her body*? This may show up as problems with the routine habits of life, such as eating, sleeping, or elimination. A youngster may have trouble controlling her bladder or regulating her bodily activity level. An adolescent may have trouble nourishing herself properly and taking pleasure in eating, so she may not eat healthily and may become very preoccupied with her appearance and weight. Despite the preceding difficulties, your child may be learning well in school and getting along well with peers.

Is your child primarily having difficulty coping with her *emotions*? Learning to manage emotions and reach out for help at the right time is a task we all work on throughout our lives. Problems may show up as a difficulty balancing particular emotions, and she may experience a great deal of sadness, anger, anxiety, or excitement. Younger children need help managing more intense emotions. Older children and adolescents must learn to take more responsibility for their feelings and discover how to seek help from others outside the family.

Despite the difficulty with particular emotions, your child may be a good student, handle other feelings well, be healthy, and have no physical symptoms. And even if she has high anxiety or depressive symptoms, she may still have good peer relationships.

Is she primarily having difficulty *forming and maintaining particular relationships*? This may show up as a problem making friendships—generally, or just with males or females. Or, she may have problems with those in authority—inside or outside the family. She may struggle to follow the rules of social custom; she may steal, lie, or bully. Commonly such problems show up when your child moves into the world and has more independent contact with others outside your family. Again, your child may be doing well in school, have many interests, take care of herself physically, and be successful in certain activities.

Last, is her difficulty mainly with *taking in and processing information*? Problems in this area show up most prominently as learning disorders, often discovered first at school. Although she may have a learning disorder, she could be doing quite well in forming relationships with peers or taking care of her body. Less common than a "simple" learning disorder, but more worrisome, your child may struggle with rational thinking or with experiencing reality as others do. This difficulty is more likely to show up in problems with relationships and managing emotions, and when severe, with managing the body.

A developmental perspective helps you remember that your child is continually changing and always growing physically and mentally. Getting physically bigger and stronger, she can go places and do things she couldn't before. Growing mentally, she can think about herself, others, and the world around her in new ways. As she grows, she also faces increasing external demands and obstacles as others' expectations of her change, and she has to cope with new situations. Each day, your child is challenged to learn new ways of dealing with different aspects of her life. These inner and outer forces propelling change may move her from a place of balance, without symptoms, to one of imbalance and disruption. Or these same forces may move her toward balance and fewer symptoms.

Using these four categories can help you see that although your child may be having a delay or disruption in one area, she may be coping successfully in other areas. Keeping a developmental perspective in mind may help you feel more compassion toward your child and yourself when things go awry. Your job requires you to help your child cope with current changes and to develop skills to cope with new changes ahead. You probably are doing this difficult job while coping with developmental changes in your own life: taking on greater work responsibilities, coping with illness or changes in your relationship with your own parents. Compassion and patience, toward yourself and your child, are useful qualities to have as you grapple with the challenging problems that inevitably come up in the job of parenting.

> Dorothy was concerned about her eight-year-old daughter, Melissa. She saw her as having no empathy or concern about anybody else's feelings. She feared that Melissa would never develop empathy. Because of her impulsivity, Melissa had been placed on medication and had responded well. However, she had lost her appetite and didn't eat as much. This had been a problem for a few months and usually Dorothy asked her daughter if she had eaten her lunch at school. On one particular day, in response to her mother's question, Melissa asked her mother if she were worried that she had not been eating as well and might lose weight. It took Dorothy some time after the conversation before she realized that her daughter was concerned about how she might be feeling. Melissa was showing empathy towards her. Dorothy also realized that she had been thinking of her daughter as static and unchanging, rather than someone who was delayed in her development and would take longer to develop certain abilities than other children her age.

Whatever your child's situation, try not to focus only on the delays and difficulties. Keep your child's strengths and accomplishments fully in mind. This will help you interact with your child in a way that helps her develop her strengths and reduce her shame and worry about her symptoms.

Infants and toddlers

Since behavioral and emotional disorders can have a physical or medical basis, *all persisting symptoms should be evaluated by a pediatrician or family practitioner.*

Disruption of bodily routine (eating, sleeping, and elimination)

From birth, your infant has the big job of transitioning successfully from living in a totally controlled environment (the womb) to living in a world where everything changes. Your infant's body must adjust to temperature changes, sound and light variations, and changing physical sensations. He must also develop patterns for taking in food, eliminating waste, and resting.

At this early stage, most disruptions have a predominantly physical basis. For example, his digestive system may find it hard to handle a particular food type and he may have a lot of gas and cramps or diarrhea, or he has an ear infection and the pain at night wakes him frequently.

However, a caretaker's own anxiety level or depression can also affect how an infant functions physically. This is especially so with very sensitive infants and toddlers, who may respond to even low levels of anxiety or depression in a mother or father.

As a parent, you naturally are invested in your newborn. When he is sick and the usual patterns of eating, sleeping, and elimination get disrupted, you feel upset and may have a hard time keeping your feelings in balance. Usually your child will heal quickly from whatever is causing illness and you will regain your emotional equilibrium. But sometimes you and your infant will get into a negative spiral: his disturbed patterns and your emotional reactions can worsen each other. To help the interaction become positive again, have an understanding family member intervene or get help from your pediatrician.

The example below shows this negative spiral in the interaction between infant and mother, and then a positive shift.

> Baby Joey had been having abdominal gas after feeding. His distress upset his first-time mother, who felt that she was doing something wrong that caused Joey's difficulty. She became quite anxious at each feeding time, and baby Joey began to reject the bottle. Her husband also became anxious. Rather than help his wife be more confident, he began to cause her worry too.
>
> The mother consulted with the pediatrician who explained that Joey might be having a hard time digesting the formula. The doctor recommended a change in formula. This relieved the mother and helped to shift the negative cycle. The mother also considered consulting a therapist to address her anxiety, but as Joey's symptom diminished with his development, the mother's anxiety disappeared.

Disruption of relationships (attachment)

Infants are hardwired to "recognize" and respond to the human face. Your older infant's smile, and his attempts to communicate with you through sound and movement, indicate that he was born with the ability to form an attachment: a trusting, positive, dependent bond. Without this kind of connection to a caregiver, an infant may not develop normally or even survive.

You may feel distressed if you do not feel connected with your infant, or if you think something is unusual in the way that your child reacts to other children or adults. Since you are naturally attuned to your child, your observations are very important. Feeling disconnected from your infant may signal subtly that he has a delay in developing his ability for social interaction or verbal and non-verbal communication.

- He may have a problem with hearing or seeing.
- He may be very sensitive or overly reactive to certain intensities of touch, sound, sight, or taste.
- He may have a problem processing (seeing and reacting to) social cues.
- He may have difficulty maintaining a consistent connection because of seizures.

If, by ten months of age, your child is not actively babbling and gesturing in response to your presence and as a way to make his wishes known, consult with a child development specialist. A complete assessment by a pediatrician or child development specialist can let you get early treatment of whatever is causing the sense of disconnection or delay. The earlier treatment is started, the better.

The next example describes how an attuned mother noticed problems early and sought intervention.

Tony was Maria's fourth child. Early on, she was pleased that he was a quiet baby who hardly ever cried. Within the first few months, she also noted that he seemed quite different from her other three children. He didn't look at her when she fed him and didn't get excited being around his siblings, as her second two babies did.

Maria and her husband shared their observations with the pediatrician, who ordered a developmental evaluation by a team of specialists. The team recommended an early intervention program to help Tony and his parents find better ways for him to cope with ordinary visual and auditory stimulation. Up to that point, the stimulation had been simply too much for his brain to handle. Tony had developed a pattern of response to slight increases in stimulation by simply "shutting down."

Through the interventions, Tony's parents learned ways to anticipate situations that would be over-stimulating for him and ways to help him develop tolerance for those situations, rather than immediately shut down.

Disruption of emotional modulation (mood, arousal, and anxiety)

Infants' moods are fairly simple. They are closely linked to their physical states of comfort or distress. Mood states largely communicate how well an infant's bodily systems—nervous system, digestive system, hormonal system, etc.—are coping with the new environment outside the womb. A child's inborn capacity for emotional states helps her become attached to caretakers and be influenced by those attachments.

A toddler's emotional states are still very connected to her physical states, yet are increasingly influenced by interactions with others. A toddler's emotional modulation (the ability to keep a positively balanced mood) is dependent upon the caretaker.

An infant or toddler may have frequent and fiery angry outbursts, intense sadness, or quiet withdrawal for many reasons.

- There may be an underlying physical problem that causes a lot of pain or discomfort.

- Your infant or toddler may have a low tolerance for the stress of change or to the loss of a comforting connection with a caretaker.

- She may have high levels of anxiety or fear caused by too much stimulation (either because the stimulation would be too much for any child, or because your child is easily over-stimulated).

- Ongoing disharmony or conflict within the family may cause your child stress. A tense environment does not support, and may undermine, a toddler's positive mood. As a result, your toddler may have a hard time handling the normal stress around transitions and may take longer to "recover" from a stressful transition or new experience.

Give your child more time for transitions, so she has time to adjust to the changes. If your child is over-stimulated, provide plenty of comforting contact, time with an important caretaker, and lots of soothing. If necessary, address the level of conflict in the family by seeking professional help.

The example below shows how an infant can respond to the emotional conflict in the adults around her and how the child's stress can diminish when the adults resolve their conflicts.

Elizabeth was just 17 years old and unmarried when she gave birth to Spencer. The new mother and son lived with the grandparents. Spencer's mother and grandmother struggled over who was the primary caretaker for Spencer. Often, after the two women had angry outbursts, the baby would wail and seem very sad and cranky. Elizabeth was taking good care of Spencer despite the tension with her own mother. As the grandmother gradually accepted that her primary role was as a support to Elizabeth and the conflict between them diminished, the baby's wailing decreased and his mood brightened.

Taking a developmental perspective on disruptions that arise in infants and toddlers will help you make better sense of what is happening since verbal communication is limited and the physical aspects of growth and change are so prominent. What is my child trying to accomplish or cope with physically? What does the symptom have to do with my child's current physical, relational, or emotional stage of development?

Preschoolers

Children aged three to five are quite responsive and reactive to their environment as well as to what might be happening between adults and them. Unlike infants and toddlers, preschoolers' disruptions will more often have psychological causes than physical ones. Nevertheless, still refer all persistent symptoms to the pediatrician, since these symptoms can certainly have medical causes.

Disruption of bodily routine (eating, sleeping, and elimination)

During the preschool years, one big achievement for children in managing their body is their ability to develop regular patterns for urinating and having bowel movements. Usually preschoolers can delay the urges to urinate or have a bowel movement, although this ability can be disrupted easily by emotional (e.g. anxiety/fear) and physical (e.g. illness) causes. Preschoolers occasionally may also have problems with eating.

Difficulty with developing proper routines for urinating and having a bowel movement are common. The most frequent symptom is bedwetting.

- Typically, bedwetting is caused by neurological immaturity, not psychological immaturity.

- Sometimes bedwetting may be the result of a regression caused by some major psychological stress, such as the birth of a sibling happening shortly after being regularly dry. A regression can also follow a physical stress, such as surgery or severe illness.

Usually, bedwetting disappears on its own as a child gets older. One in five children aged five years wet the bed; one in twenty by age ten; and one or two in one hundred by age 15 (see Chapter 2, **Wetting**).

Problems with bowel habits come about for many reasons:

- Typically, bowel problems occur in a child who is somewhat immature emotionally and socially.

- Immature children are more vulnerable to stresses that can interfere with developing good toileting routines.

- Specific stresses include the absence of a parent from the household (such as a father on military duty overseas).

- A parent and child may develop conflict about when or where the child should have a bowel movement. At that point control and power become the main forces in the relationship, rather than the child's wish to please and stay attached to the parent.

- Rarely, the colon may have an abnormality in how it works.

Your child's main motive in learning to delay the urge to urinate or have a bowel movement in the toilet is to please you. Thus, fostering a loving relationship with your preschooler will help him want to take on these routines.

Your child will get bowel control, on *his* timetable. Although he may be having a problem, notice all the other things he is doing well. Get professional help early so a relatively short-term difficulty does not become a longer-term problem (see Chapter 2, **Soiling**).

The example below illustrates how one mother shifted the power struggle with her daughter to a more positive and cooperative approach to toilet training.

Veronica, who recently turned five, was in an intense struggle with her mother around bowel movements. She did not use the bathroom at daycare and would frequently hold her stool in for several days. Early on in her toilet training, Veronica held her bowel movements so long that it hurt a great deal when she finally did sit on the toilet.

She would keep herself from having a bowel movement for a long time, and then eventually would lose control of her stool. She would soil her underpants. Her mom had her use diapers, largely out of frustration about what else to do. Because Veronica refused to use the toilet, she also often got stomach aches that required her to use an enema.

Her mother tried both simple explaining and angry yelling. Neither approach kept Veronica from holding her stool in. When someone asked Veronica if she had to use the potty, she regularly would shake her curly blond head, "No." Sometimes Veronica's mother could get her daughter to sit on the toilet after meals on a regular basis. But, after a while, the pattern would be broken because neither of them could maintain a consistent balanced approach.

Summertime came. Veronica wanted to go to camp and swim. Her mother began threatening that she would not send her if she did not "do your stinkies in the toilet." This just inflamed their conflict. I suggested to Veronica's mother that she clearly explain the camp rule to Veronica: only children who were toilet trained could use the swimming pool. Veronica's mother told her daughter that she would let her go to camp but that the staff wouldn't let her use the swimming pool because she still wasn't toilet trained. She offered to help Veronica so that she would be able to use the swimming pool. She became Veronica's advocate instead of her barrier. With this change in relationship, Veronica and her mother developed a plan so that she regularly used the toilet, stopped soiling, and was able to go to camp and use the swimming pool.

Like other preschoolers, Veronica was working to acquire some control of her own body. Because of the painful experience when she first began to use the toilet, she was frightened and wanted to withdraw from the task. She preferred to avoid the whole problem. At first her mother got caught up in her daughter's fear and tried to control Veronica (both her fear and her bowel movements). The situation improved when Veronica's mother got control of her own fear and helped her daughter see the positive advantages of being in better control of her bowel movements. Veronica then easily moved beyond her delay in this developmental task.

Disruption of bodily activity (movement)

Your preschooler is a bundle of energy and "in love with" the world. There is so much that is new. At this age, action seems to be the primary way of engaging with the world, just as "mouthing" was for your infant. Your child's ability to delay activity and manage impulses usually grows quite a bit during this developmental period. It has to develop so that formal schooling can take place during the next phase of growing up.

Some children who have an abnormally high level of activity may first be identified as "overactive" by a preschool teacher, especially if the children have had some socialization experiences with other children in daycare. Such children may not be identified as "abnormally hyperactive" (meaning they would be diagnosed with attention deficit hyperactivity disorder (ADHD)) until they start elementary school. This may be because there is a high tolerance for activity in kindergarten, the hyperactivity is only of a moderate level (and manageable when children don't have to spend long periods of time sitting), or the child can follow rules well enough that he doesn't present with a behavior problem when there are consistent rules and good structure.

If your child is hyperactive (whether or not he gets a diagnosis of ADHD), make sure he has plenty of physical outlets as well as firm and kind guidance and limits for his impulsive side. This will give him the time to gain better control of his activity level and impulses, and minimize the chances that he will form a negative self-image from having his high energy and impulsivity get him into trouble.

For a child under six, who is considered hyperactive, medication is only used occasionally since it is often hard to distinguish normal high activity from problematic hyperactivity.

Some children, who at first seem to be simply hyperactive, may have other issues present:

- They may be easily hyper-aroused by anxiety or other strong emotions that go along with ordinary stress, or they may be chronically over-aroused by extraordinary family stress. (If your child is overactive in just one setting, or just occasionally, this is more likely to be due to anxiety, not just hyperactivity and inattention.)

- There may be delays in other aspects of your child's development. For example, he may be delayed in language development or in his social–emotional development.

Hypoactivity (under-activity) may also be present in this age group and has several likely causes:

- physical illness that comes on suddenly, or ongoing problems like asthma or chronic infections
- depression
- other problems in development that need to be evaluated.

The example below describes a child who struggled with hyperactivity, and shows how his mother and daycare providers cooperated to give him more structure and support.

> The daycare staff called Jeff's mom to tell her that he was on the verge of being kicked out. Apparently he was continually getting into conflict with the staff. He was not listening when they wanted him to sit quietly and pay attention to a story that was being read aloud. They wanted him to play quietly at the art table and be able to settle down and take a nap like the other children. He was always moving around, talking to the child next to him during story time, and unable to rest silently at nap period. Sometimes the conflicts would escalate.
>
> Jeff would have crying tantrums and the staff would get annoyed. Jeff's mother asked a consultant to evaluate the situation. The consultant spent a few mornings observing Jeff in the daycare. She concluded that at some point Jeff, who was four years old, could be diagnosed as having ADHD, but that he might be just a somewhat overly exuberant four-year-old.
>
> She recommended that Jeff have closer supervision, as he could easily become over-stimulated. This meant that he would sit next to the teacher during story time, have a staff person next to him at the art table, and be set up for a nap in an area away from the other children. She also suggested to the daycare center staff that they have an outdoor activity for the children just before they did a quiet activity. She had noticed that Jeff (and some other children) seemed calmer after they got to play outside. These changes resulted in less conflict between the staff and Jeff. His tantrums ended.

Disruption of emotional modulation (mood, arousal, and anxiety)

Your preschooler's emotional experience has all the ingredients found in an adult's emotional repertoire, including envy, jealousy, shame, guilt, love, hate, joy, fear, and courage. But your child's ability to balance, or modulate, emotional experience has much more development and growth to come.

Preschoolers can have the full scope of adult emotional difficulties, although often in a simpler or slightly different form. Anxiety (excessive fear) and depression (prolonged sadness or irritability) can certainly be present in your child at this age. Usually these emotional states do not last very long. Sleep difficulties can be an early sign of a developing disruption of emotional modulation. A high level of fear or sadness may come up for several reasons:

- Your child may be highly sensitive to ordinary stress and change.
- Your child may be responding to major disruptive events, such as the death of a parent, divorce, hospitalization, surgery, traumatic accidents, or abuse.

Medications are rarely used for preschoolers, largely because children are often quite responsive to environmental changes and the mood states are often time-limited. Psychological or social interventions are most often carried out with the family and caretakers, although occasionally with the child directly.

The example below illustrates how intense emotions often have underlying psychological causes that can be addressed.

> Five-year-old Stephen had begun having difficulty in daycare and at home. When in the midst of a tantrum, he would often bite himself or try to hit his mother or throw something at her. The oldest of three children, Stephen had not seen his father for four months. His father was an alcoholic who frequently had rage attacks. He had been physically abusive to Stephen's mother and had disappeared after a particularly violent outburst.
>
> The daycare staff found that Stephen's tantrums were less intense when he was around one of the male staff who could nurture and gently roughhouse with him, and give Stephen firm and kind limits, especially regarding his "angry energy." As Stephen's involvement with this particular male staff grew, Stephen's behavior at home also began to improve.
>
> Stephen had experienced many losses and frustrations for his young age. His anger had been over-stimulated. Little boys at his age are just beginning to learn to be assertive and to express anger appropriately when they don't like something, and need a male figure to model how to express appropriately and tolerate such feelings. Fortunately, Stephen found one at daycare.

Disruption of relationships (attachment)

The variety of relationships that an older preschooler may have can resemble those of school-aged children. There are buddies, rivals, heroes, etc. These relationships are strongly influenced by the child's emotions; consequently, preschoolers do not usually have long-lasting connections and interests in others. Your preschooler is just beginning to develop the ability to keep a connection with another person in the face of negative emotions, such as fear, anger, and sadness. It is far more limited now than it will be when he is a school-aged child.

A child with relationship difficulties may be shy, avoiding verbal, physical, or social interaction. Or he may indiscriminately approach perfect strangers. He might be strongly oppositional and defiant (especially with authority figures) and have a hard time keeping a positive connection to caretakers. None of these patterns predicts what your son or daughter will be like as an older child or adolescent, or as an adult.

Many factors contribute to problems with relationships at this age:

- Your child may have a hard time keeping emotional balance.
- Your child may be hyperactive, which makes it hard for him to make and keep comforting connections.
- Your child may have attachment difficulties because of many past disrupted connections.

You can take steps to keep your child's unusual or extreme patterns of relating from becoming more extreme or habitual. Some children, because of earlier traumatic experiences or their great sensitivity, experience intense feelings when first interacting with another person.

- Help your child find ways to express and cope with the fear, shame, or anger that may come up for him in connections with others.
- Let your child know that it is okay to feel scared, angry, or embarrassed, and that there are acceptable and unacceptable ways to express such feelings.
- Talk about what your child is feeling in a non-judgmental manner.
- Consider giving explicit suggestions about how to respond and behave in a given situation. A child who feels understood is usually open to hearing such practical suggestions.

As children grow and cope better with difficult feelings, their relationships can improve. The example below illustrates how one couple helped their daughter cope with her fear in new social situations.

Samantha was very talkative when with her immediate family. However, whenever a stranger, or someone she knew just a little bit, came to her house, she hardly spoke. In daycare, she never spoke to the teacher directly, and just shook her head yes or no. Her parents were surprised by her behavior, since she seemed somewhat fearless when playing on the jungle gym or learning to ride her bike.

They began to understand that she experienced a great deal of fear and shame in new social situations. They took steps to help her cope with those strong feelings. Her parents spent extra time in the daycare while she was there, and invited the teacher to visit their home, hoping that would make her seem more like an immediate family member and safer for Samantha.

Samantha's parents found that it did not help to ask Samantha what she felt when she was around others. But when they non-judgmentally said what they *thought* she might be feeling, she passed through her distressed states more quickly. As time passed, she also began to use their words to describe her experience.

Preschoolers, especially aged four to five, sometimes may seem like "little adults" as they engage with the challenges of coping with their emotions and relationships with others. Hold on to a developmental perspective so you do not overestimate your child's abilities and can make better sense of the difficulties that you and she run into.

School-aged children: 6–12
Disruption of bodily routine (eating, sleeping, and elimination)

By the time children begin school, most have firmly established the routines of eating, sleeping, and elimination, although turbulent emotional states and troublesome relationships may disrupt those routines. Normal patterns can vary. For example, a child may like or dislike particular foods, have a special routine for getting to sleep, and show some quirks around toileting habits.

If your child still has persistent problems with bedwetting or soiling by this age, it can impact on his social life, self-image, and emotional development. Continued bedwetting is likely to be due to delayed body maturation. Be patient and supportive, and consider medication if bedwetting makes your child feel too self-conscious to want to sleep over with peers (see Chapter 9 on medication treatment).

If your child is still soiling his underwear with feces, there are likely to be several other areas of difficulty:

- Your child may be having a hard time engaging in relationships with others.
- He may be having difficulty managing emotions in a balanced way.
- He may need more support and structure to learn how to manage his body properly.

If your child is still soiling himself by age six, consult with a pediatrician or specialist. The story below illustrates some of the underlying causes for soiling (disrupted training, immaturity, social isolation), and how one mother, with the help of a doctor, identified physical, social, and psychological ways to help her son.

Ten-year-old Brian had been soiling his underwear with fecal matter since he began school. Although he was toilet trained by age five, he went through phases when he would soil his underwear and hide it in his bedroom. His mother would find the soiled underwear hidden in the closet or under the bed. Sometimes a teacher would tell Brian's mother that Brian smelled bad.

Brian's mother wasn't sure what to do to help her son. A single parent since Brian was about four, she worked days. She felt embarrassed that he had never stayed fully toilet trained. She wasn't sure how much his difficulty making friends contributed to his problem and how much it was the result of his problem. Generally he seemed unhappy, with little interest in outside activities. He would often spend time after school watching television and eating junk food.

At her wits' end, she overcame her embarrassment and consulted the family pediatrician. The doctor put Brian on a proper diet and a regimen of stool softeners; he also planned set times for Brian to sit on the toilet. Brian's mother provided support by writing out the whole plan and offering Brian incentives if he stuck to the program.

The doctor also encouraged Brian's mother to arrange for her son to be in an after-school program three days a week and to have an older adolescent companion to do activities with Brian on the other weekdays. The doctor also suggested the local Big Brothers/Big Sisters program as another resource.

Brian's mother had thought her son was responsible enough to take care of himself without getting into trouble, which was true. But she had not fully considered his need for structured social experiences. Although Brian did reasonably well in school, he was emotionally and socially immature and needed extra support in those arenas. With the added structure and social engagement, Brian's mood improved. He began to show a genuine interest in peers and his toileting problem faded away.

In retrospect it appears that Brian was stuck in a younger developmental stage which required his mother to provide closer monitoring and guidance than she had realized. When he got that better oversight, he began to "catch up with himself."

Disruption of bodily activity (movement)

A school-aged child's ability to delay impulsive behavior (stoked by excitement, desire, or the need to avoid emotional pain) has improved considerably over the preschooler's. Children of this age are better at voluntarily controlling complex muscle movements, which means they can participate in sports and arts. Their attention span has also lengthened. While at times the expectations and demands of adults exceed a child's ability to "listen, sit still, be quiet," most times, the child can do so.

Problems with hyperactivity, impulsivity, and attention span are thought to be mainly due to an immaturity in the development of the brain areas related to the ability to delay reacting. There are several possible causes.

- The immaturity and delay in development may be inherited.

- It may be due to a prenatal or early life insult to the brain, such as an infection or drug use during pregnancy.

- A biological tendency (caused by one of the above) may be magnified by chronic over-stimulation (like too much visual or emotional stimulation), not enough structure and routine that is calming, or a hypersensitivity to certain foods or chemicals.

If a child's activity level, attention span, and level of impulsivity remain immature, it can be harder for him to perform in school and get along with peers. Imagine if you went to work each day and your supervisor criticized your performance. You couldn't figure out how to make it better on your own, and your fellow workers rolled their eyes at how you behaved. This might be the internal experience of your child who is coping with problems of hyperactivity, inattention/distractibility and impulsivity (ADHD) in the school setting.

If your child's school work and relationships with others are not going well, the pediatrician or mental health specialist (after considering all the possibilities and perhaps seeking a psychological evaluation) might recommend medication (see

Chapter 2, **Inattention** and **Hyperactivity**; Chapter 6, "A. Psychological tests," and Chapter 9).

The following example describes how a young boy's parents recognized his immaturity and intervened to be sure he got the support he needed to succeed in school.

> José started fourth grade as a happy and friendly little boy who preferred recess and active play to class work. He got along with his classmates and teacher but was falling behind in reading and math skills. During class, he chatted with the students around him and had a hard time paying attention to the teacher. The other students liked him but complained that José always wanted to talk with them while they were trying to work.
>
> José told his parents that he didn't like going to school since he always got in trouble. His parents were aware that he was somewhat immature, so decided to talk with the teacher. After the meeting, the teacher moved José to a desk in front of the room, on an end aisle. She also arranged for him to have one-on-one help with his academic work and made sure that he was paying attention to her as she spoke to the whole class. Gradually, José complained less about school and talked more about the classmates he liked and his accomplishments in reading and math.

A child in this age group may have a kind of disruption in bodily movement not seen in the younger groups: tics. It is not uncommon for school-aged children, especially around age ten, to have brief, infrequent, and repetitive twitches or tics of the muscles in their upper body, neck, and head. The cause of such excessive movement is not understood, but one theory is that it is linked to increased anxiety that comes with a greater social consciousness. Such tic movements pass after a few weeks but sometimes remain. Longer lasting motor tics may be accompanied by "vocal tics," such as coughing, clearing the throat, or making noises and then be formally diagnosed as Tourette's syndrome (see Chapter 2, **Tics**).

Disruption of emotional modulation (mood, arousal, and anxiety)

School-aged children are actively engaged in developing more sophisticated methods to cope with and manage emotional experience. Secrets, private fantasies, and deeper feelings all are now possible. This adds a layer of complexity to your child's life that enriches it and also makes it more stressful.

While anxiety is a part of every child's life, for some it can be disruptively high. If your child has a high level of anxiety, it may appear as fear or worry connected to a specific situation (such as a fear of the dark or of meeting new people). Anxiety can also show up before or after whatever triggered the fear. For example, your school-aged child may dawdle or make excuses to avoid some place that makes him anxious. Or he may obsess about a situation and engage in magical rituals before or after some particular event or experience. This is in contrast to the preschooler or young school-aged child who may experience anxiety only when immediately confronting the triggering situation.

Your child may also remain unhappy longer than he did when younger. His unhappiness may dominate his daily mood and behavior; he may even seem depressed. As your child becomes more self-aware, he also may start to express anger with himself for being unhappy. This stance may exist side by side with an earlier coping style of being angry with others for "causing" his unhappiness (see Chapter 2, **Depression** or **Anxiety**).

Recently, professionals in the child mental health field have paid a lot of attention to children who have intense periods of irritability or great mood swings. Some experts think that these children have an early form of bipolar disorder. But since the mix of the causes will most likely be unique to your child, I believe that there should be caution in labeling a child with a specific diagnosis of bipolar disorder. The term is usually used to imply a lifelong disorder from largely biological causes; but with many school-aged children, it is not clear that the cause is primarily biological, especially when there is no family history of bipolar disorder. It just makes things more stressful to imply that your child has a lifelong disorder when that may not be so.

We do not understand all the causes of bipolar type mood disorder but we do know that children often have trouble balancing their mood states due to interacting factors:

- The child's temperament may make him very sensitive and intensely reactive to frustration, embarrassment, or fear.

- This may be magnified because the child has not yet learned how to cope with such intensity.

- The child may have been through excessively stressful or abusive life experiences, which continually bring up intense emotion.

- The child may not have had enough modeling for how to cope with intense or painful emotions.

The example below shows how a child with disruptive anxiety, triggered by the experience of multiple losses in her life, moved past her difficulty.

Amanda, a conscientious and recently somewhat somber third-grader, was nine when she began to ask her mother about health matters. At first her mother didn't see anything unusual. However, her daughter began to ask the same question repetitively, often before bed. "Are there lots of germs on the doorknobs in school?" "Can I get sick and die from touching the doorknobs in school?" "Could I pass those germs on to you and could you get sick and die from them?"

Her mother first tried to reassure Amanda, but that didn't help much. Her mother consulted with the pediatrician. He asked if Amanda experienced compulsive rituals that sometimes accompany obsessive thoughts. Her mother found out that indeed Amanda tried to avoid touching doorknobs and washed her hands repetitively if she did touch knobs. The pediatrician recommended a psychotherapist for Amanda. Amanda only went twice: she said she didn't find it helpful and didn't want to talk with the therapist anymore.

Amanda's mother continued to meet with the therapist on her own. She came to understand that her daughter had a number of recent stresses that contributed to her high level of anxiety. Amanda's second-grade teacher had died suddenly in the middle of the school year. Three months later, her maternal grandfather died. She had been close with both people, yet seemed rather restrained and precociously mature in dealing with those deaths. Amanda's mother also realized that she had been somewhat withdrawn from her daughter as a result of her own prolonged grief after the death of her father, Amanda's grandfather.

Amanda's mother began to respond to her daughter's questions more as expressions of her emotional struggles than as a search for "facts." She also began to see how anxious her daughter was. She encouraged her daughter to tolerate the anxiety of not doing the rituals and find other ways to cope. She worked with Amanda on this task and became more emotionally engaged with her daughter.

Amanda's mood became lighter. She was less compulsive about her studies and more involved with her peers. Her persistent questions slowly faded away. Amanda's mother had learned that medication might help her daughter's symptoms, but since the symptoms had practically disappeared, she decided not to pursue that avenue.

Amanda was more aware of life's unpredictability because of her experience with the death of people close to her and her mother's relative absence in response to the grandfather's death. Left alone to cope with the emotions and her over-stimulated imagination, Amanda got stuck. When her mother became more emotionally available and put into action what she had learned from the therapist, Amanda got unstuck. Amanda's mood improved and she became more socially engaged with peers.

Disruption of relationships (attachment)

By this age, coping with relationships within the family has generally become routine. The arena for social exploration and development now largely involves peers. Special friends, buddies, crushes, and team mates are all now possible. These kinds of connections are very important for the development of emotional and social skills. Once again, these wider social experiences enrich life as well as make it much more complicated.

You may notice that your child is having problems in this area because he has no friends or tends to be excessively disappointed, angry, or fearful with others. Your child might have a problem with everyone outside of the family or just with specific outsiders (such as just peers, just adults, just with males, or just with females). In school-aged children several inter-related factors may cause problems with relationships:

- Relationship difficulties may be influenced by your child's inborn temperament. For example, your child may quickly get very shy or intensely anxious when with people.

- There may be some specific deficiency, such as a problem with making sense of social cues or understanding complex social situations. If so, he may quickly be overwhelmed or confused in new situations.

- There may be stressful early life experiences, such as an unendingly bitter divorce, domestic violence, medical ordeals like surgery or multiple hospitalizations, or experiences of physical or sexual abuse, which undermine a sense of trust and safety.

- Most commonly, relationship problems are due to a combination of the preceding causes.

Ongoing problems with connections to others are a part of many formal psychiatric diagnoses, ranging from oppositional defiant disorder and social phobia to pervasive developmental disorder, high functioning autism subtype. Children with such problems must learn how to:

- feel safe with another person

- figure out how much to trust another person

- find how to tolerate disappointment and not give up trying to form relationships.

The example below describes how one mother helped her child maintain her connections with her peers.

Amanda (described in an earlier vignette) also had disruptions in her attachments after her teacher and grandfather died. She had stopped going to friends' houses for sleep-overs and had become somewhat irritable and aloof with classmates. She complained to her mother that "no one is my friend."

Amanda's problems were an exaggeration of a situation that had occurred in kindergarten, when she first started school, but seemed to have faded during the first and second grades. In fact, Amanda was quite actively involved with her classmates during the earlier part of the school year, before her second-grade teacher died. In kindergarten, Amanda had been shy and easily disappointed when an overture she made to a classmate was not reciprocated. Her mother remembered that Amanda occasionally came home from kindergarten unhappy, reporting that she hadn't played with anyone during the free play time. At that time, Amanda's mother spoke with the teacher who then made an extra effort to foster connections between Amanda and some other kindergartners.

Making some new efforts to help her daughter, Amanda's mother suggested that her daughter host a sleep-over with some classmates. She also encouraged Amanda to invite a friend to join the family for dinner or a weekend trip.

Amanda had had a sensitivity to feeling rejected that preceded the deaths of her teacher and grandfather. Her mother helped her overcome her tendency to withdraw and feel excluded when she provided Amanda with extra support to form and maintain connections with friends.

Disruption of relationships (social custom)

Many rules, routines, and traditions based on gender, social class, ethnic grouping, etc. become established during children's school-aged years. Children must learn a great deal about how to interact with others, some of which is taught directly and some of which they must take in intuitively. Some children are better at learning social rules and customs than others. Stable and secure family relationships allow your child to give full attention to this task outside the home.

This type of disruption includes behaviors (such as lying, cheating, stealing, and other antisocial activities) which may not seem to distress your child, but can distress you and others around your child. Your son may see the adults' distress as the problem, rather than his own behavior or internal states.

The causes for such behaviors vary, depending in part on the age of your child.

- A younger school-aged child may lie or cheat because he has not developed better ways to manage the fear, disappointment, and anger connected with a social situation.

- At a young age, the behavior is unlikely to be out of a habitual pattern. Such behavior is like taking a "shortcut": a child might lie or steal to get something quickly that he wants very badly. Or he may lie to avoid a negative consequence, such as a parent's anger or a restriction from television, which he does not know how to cope with or tolerate.

- Younger school-aged children may also engage in antisocial or destructive behavior to "belong" to a peer group. Your child might lie, cheat, steal, etc. because he's seen siblings, peers, older friends or adults do it.

- A child's worrisome behavior might also be connected to ongoing family stress or a failure to learn basic social norms.

- Your child may also have an ongoing mood disruption, such as a depression, which leaves him with a low tolerance for frustration and a high need for stimulation and pleasure.

- Your child may only connect weakly with others and may not emotionally experience how his behavior harms others.

- Your child may be impulsive and steal without being able to think through the consequences of his action.

- For older children, the use of alcohol or drugs might further contribute to lying and stealing.

- (See Chapter 2, **Cheating**, **Lying**, **Stealing**, and **Oppositional behavior**.)

Unsociable behavior may have only one main cause: more often, it has many. As your son moves from earlier (ages 6–8) to later (ages 9–12) childhood, he may develop a repetitive pattern of oppositional and antisocial behavior as his primary style of inter-acting (see Chapter 2, **Oppositional behaviour**).

The example below illustrates how one family gradually acknowledged and addressed the stresses that were causing their son to engage in antisocial behavior.

Dennis was about to begin junior high school. He had not expressed any worry about leaving his elementary school of six years, but during the summer before seventh grade he began hanging out at the mall with some older boys his parents did not know. His parents noticed that his attitude and language towards them had become slightly disrespectful. One time his parents noted that he was wearing clothing that they had not bought him. He said that the clothes were ones that he had traded with one of his new friends. A few days later, the family got a call from a clothing store at the mall saying that their son had been caught shoplifting.

The parents paid for the clothes and told Dennis they were taking it out of his allowance. He also had to write a letter of apology to the clothing store owner and was banned from the mall for one year. His parents put him in a day camp program for the rest of the summer. They also talked with him about starting junior high school. They explained that he would have a lot of structure with regard to homework time, and strict limits with regard to Internet, instant messaging, and video game time. While Dennis protested, his parents thought that he seemed much less erratic and irritable, and more respectful.

His father, who had started a new job that summer and was quite preoccupied, made an effort to do extra activities with Dennis. He tried to respond positively when Dennis took a more active role doing chores around the house without conflict. Dennis's father encouraged him to invite some of his elementary school friends, whom his father knew, to join them when they were going to a professional baseball game and to an amusement park.

Dennis was in the midst of a big transition from elementary school to junior high. While his parents had initially given him some extra freedom, they quickly realized that he needed extra guidance and support during the transition, not less.

Disruption of information processing (learning)

The school setting is an arena for developing and practicing relationship skills, especially during the elementary years. However, the main task is to take in information about the world and to develop and strengthen the capacity for logical thought.

Your child may not learn school material at the rate expected of her (compared to other children her age or to what is seen as her overall potential or intelligence). Disruptions in learning may first come to light because of behavioral problems at school. Such behaviors, caused by an underlying learning disorder, often show up when a child is in the first or second grade, although sometimes not until later.

If there are no behavioral troubles that call attention to an underlying learning problem, then such a problem may be identified later, usually as a result of failing test scores. This often happens in the third grade when the amount and complexity of school work increases. Yet, if your child is intellectually advanced or if the school staff doesn't pick up on the signs, learning problems may not be identified until later.

Problems with learning may be contributed to by other types of disruptions that prevent your daughter from taking in what is taught in the regular school setting:

- Problems with attention or emotional difficulties (like depression) may disrupt learning.

- Specific sensory problems (such as visual or hearing impairments) may disrupt the processing of information.

- Your child's brain may have a distinctive way of taking in, processing, and putting into speech or writing visual and auditory information. This problem is referred to as a "specific learning disorder." It is different from an overall slowness in all learning that comes from a generalized low intelligence. Specific learning disorders and attentional problems commonly occur together.

Examples of specific learning disorders include the following: dyslexia (reading disorder), expressive or receptive language disorders (speaking or understanding intelligibly), and visual–motor integration difficulties (hand–eye coordination, as in writing). Learning problems that show up as difficulties with planning, organizing, carrying out, and completing a task are referred to as "disorders of executive function." They are often associated with problems with attention. A comprehensive evaluation by a psychologist or a neuropsychologist may be needed to clarify if this difficulty exists and if so, why (see Chapter 6 for more information on the evaluation of a learning disorder).

Especially when unidentified, specific learning disorders can cause your child a lot of stress in school, which in turn may lead to behavioral and emotional problems. Of course, the development of additional behavioral and emotional troubles further complicates the overall difficulty with learning.

The example below illustrates how one family became aware of, and helped, their son address his learning difficulties.

Dennis (from an earlier vignette) had had a hard time with sixth grade mathematics, although he had been identified as a bright boy. His parents were both teachers, so he felt some pressure to do well in school. He had masked his embarrassment about not being able to do well at math by being a class clown and was often testy with his mathematics teacher. He frequently misplaced his math homework. If he did the homework (which was unlikely to happen if one of his parents didn't closely monitor and coach him) he did not hand it in. Given that Dennis seemed to be a bright boy who did well in English and social studies, his teacher and his parents thought that Dennis "just didn't try hard enough."

The school psychologist suggested testing for the presence of a learning disorder. To everyone's surprise, it turned out that Dennis indeed had a specific problem with processing mathematical symbols and concepts. However, even more to everyone's surprise, Dennis was identified as having evidence of an attention disorder. It seemed that his learning problems in math were further complicated by his difficulty sustaining attention. Because he did not have any difficulty with English and social studies, his problem with attention was not as evident there.

Dennis's parents got a math tutor for him and arranged for someone to help him with his math homework at school. The teacher put Dennis in the front row of class to maximize his ability to keep his attention focused. His parents monitored his math homework and communicated regularly with the mathematics teacher. Dennis's parents spoke with the pediatrician about a trial on stimulant medication for his attentional difficulties, but decided to see if the extra structure was sufficient to help him get back on track before trying medication.

There are often many reasons contributing to a particular disruption in a school-aged child. Keeping a developmental perspective helps you decide what levels of help—biologically, psychologically, socially and educationally—your child needs to move beyond the particular symptom/block in development.

Adolescents

Disruption of bodily routine (eating, sleeping, and elimination)

As puberty begins, your child must cope with a body that is getting bigger and changing dramatically. The bodily habits of eating and sleeping that he developed over the preceding decade are now up for revision. And since your child is also maturing psychologically and sexually, these everyday behaviors take on added meanings. Not only may your child have an increased appetite, but also new concerns about his body's size, shape, strength, and general appearance. Your child's sleep patterns can become erratic, because of physiological, psychological, and social changes. Adolescents must develop new self-care habits to address recently developed bodily odors, hair, and skin eruptions. The genital area, which used to be mostly related to elimination, now becomes associated with sexual excitement and relationships. All these changes, plus the habits developed to deal with them, ultimately affect your adolescent's maturing self-image and relationships with others.

Only a small percentage of adolescents continue to have problems like wetting the bed or soiling themselves. If either is present, it is likely to be a sign of a serious disruption in mood modulation or thinking.

More commonly, adolescents show disruptions in bodily habits through lapses in self-grooming, such as infrequently showering, not changing dirty clothes, etc. These lapses often happen when an adolescent feels overwhelmed with the burden of caring for himself and are usually brief and temporary. If ongoing, such symptoms may represent more serious disruptions in mood (depression) or thinking (paranoid withdrawal).

At this age, problems with getting enough sleep are common. Several typical causes of this problem fall under the heading of "poor sleep hygiene":

- Your child may get highly distracted and over-stimulated right before bed by talking on the telephone or instant messaging on the computer.

- He may fail to develop calming and soothing routines for falling asleep.

- He may have erratic bedtimes rather than developing reasonable, regular, and predictable "lights out" and wake up times.

- Your child may also have high levels of anxiety or be depressed.

For adolescent girls in particular, eating disorders become prominent after puberty. Such problems may be either a passing phase or an early stage in a serious disorder. Family therapy within the first year of the appearance of the eating disorder can help (see Chapter 2, **Eating disorders**).

The story below illustrates how a teenage girl can develop unhealthy eating and exercise patterns in an attempt to manage difficult emotions.

Martha had been a very diligent student in high school and was now a senior. She had put enormous effort into her school work and was accepted at a prestigious college. While applying to college, she had dealt with her anxiety by eating junk food. Having put on ten pounds over that period, she decided to lose it. Her mother was delighted, since she had thought that Martha was overweight and had criticized her about it for many years.

Martha undertook dieting and exercise with the same diligence she had shown about her school work. Six weeks later she had lost the ten pounds and said she wanted to lose ten more. Her mother, who had been preoccupied with her own weight off and on during her life, thought Martha's idea was "terrific."

After another six weeks and the loss of ten more pounds, Martha started to talk about losing still ten more. Her mother began to worry. Martha had increased her exercise and cut down more on what she was eating. When Martha's mother addressed this, Martha got irritated. She said that she felt fine, but thought she was still fat. This comment distressed her mother, since Martha had started looking gaunt. A friend of Martha's mother had asked her if her daughter was "anorexic."

During this whole time, Martha had never said anything about the fact that she would be leaving home and going off to college soon or how she felt about that transition. For that matter, she didn't say much of how she felt about anything. Martha had become withdrawn and quite self-absorbed.

Martha's mother took her to the family pediatrician, who found that Martha was now about 15 percent underweight. She was obsessed with her exercise program, what she ate, how much she weighed, and how fat she looked. Martha acknowledged that she felt she had "lost control" of her dieting, even though a part of her wanted to continue.

The pediatrician recommended a local 12-step program for girls with eating disorders and planned to monitor her weight over the next two months. He knew the family and the fact that the transition of Martha's leaving home would be hard for all of them, since Martha was an only child. He sensed that Martha's eating disorder was linked in some way to this transition. He recommended family therapy to help them cope better.

Disruption of bodily activity (movement)

Early adolescents naturally go through periods of high activity. Such times are linked to the bodily changes and are further fueled by the exciting sexual tone that relationships take on. Your child may have periods of great activity that alternate with periods of tiredness and lack of energy. Such natural phases of sluggishness may represent periods of temporary withdrawal from the turmoil of pubescent and adolescent life; they provide an opportunity for recovery and renewal.

During the teenage years, children with ADHD generally get less hyperactive, although they may still be very physical or fidgety. Yet problems with attention and impulsivity frequently remain, and adolescents often still need medication to manage these problems. Medication may also have a positive effect on problems with organization. Stimulant medication generally continues to be effective into adulthood for lasting problems with attention.

Being treated with medication for hyperactivity and poor attention does *not* predispose an adolescent to using recreational drugs. In fact, some research indicates that medication may actually decrease the likelihood of substance abuse for children and adolescents with hyperactivity, impulsivity, and attention problems. This may have something to do with their higher level of success than those untreated and the improved decision making because of decreased impulsivity. The severity of your child's poor attention, impulsivity, and organizational difficulties, as well as his willingness to accept responsibility for coping with his problems, influence whether or not medication continues into adolescence and beyond.

The story below illustrates how one young man used medication to help with his attention problems, while also developing other ways to cope.

Charles was looking forward to college. He had never found the work in high school particularly difficult. As a younger boy he was physically very active and found that doing a sport each season helped him manage his high energy level. While he was not terribly well organized and tended to put off studying for an exam until the last minute, he nevertheless did well enough to get into a good college.

During the first semester of his sophomore year in college, his grades went down. He noticed that it took him a lot longer to complete his assignments and study for exams than his friends. He had thought this was because he spent time chatting with peers. But even when he removed himself from distractions, he still took longer to complete the difficult assignments.

He sought help at the school counseling center. They recommended psychological testing. It turned out that Charles had a mild attention deficit disorder that affected his ability to complete large and difficult assignments in a timely fashion.

He was conflicted about using medication as he wanted to do the work "on my own." But he decided to use medication at the end of the semester when the workload and time pressures were the most intense. At other times, with his new understanding about his difficulty, he structured his study time so that there were no distractions for several hours each evening. While it still took him longer to complete his work than it might have with medication, he found that regularly structuring his time helped considerably.

Charles might not have run into his difficulty if he did not have a mild attention deficit disorder or if he had not taken a very difficult academic load that so taxed his abilities.

Disruption of emotional modulation (mood, arousal, and anxiety)

The changes that take place in adolescence stir up a lot of emotion. Internally there is a major physical and psychological makeover. Externally there is a great increase in the complexity of relationships and social roles. Passionate engagement in relationships with other people, with ideas, and with particular activities or interests is a hallmark of adolescence. It is small wonder that your adolescent may show a rise in moodiness and emotional sensitivity.

One common disruption of emotional modulation in an adolescent is depression, which may look a lot like it does in an adult. Symptoms can include:

- excessive sadness and self-critical thoughts
- excessive sleep or difficulty sleeping
- excessive eating or absence of appetite
- loss of interest in usual activities
- problems doing or getting to work (school)
- suicidal thoughts.

Psychological causes of depression in adolescents commonly fall into three areas:

- trouble giving up earlier childhood roles and gratifications
- the presence of an unresolved conflict-filled relationship, often within the family, but also outside
- some relationship loss that is not adequately grieved (such as the death of a family member with whom a very conflicted relationship existed or a love relationship that didn't work out).

If your adolescent tries to cope with a serious depression without help, it may lead to other ways of acting or feeling that take on a "life of their own." For example:

- Your adolescent may use alcohol or drugs as "medication" in an attempt to avoid feeling depressed.

- Your adolescent may develop a pattern of angry explosive behavior to avoid intolerable feelings of disappointment or worry.

- Your adolescent may become preoccupied with body image; this may distract from, and at the same time express, such painful feelings as shame, fear, or despair. That is, while the despair, shame, or fear may come from other aspects of your teenager's life, she might experience such feelings as all "due to" her appearance and become very preoccupied with her body.

- Your adolescent may purposefully injur herself in an attempt to ward off, and express, despair, fear, anger, or shame (see Chapter 2, **Self-injury/ Self-abuse**). While such behavior may be picked up by hearing about other teens doing it (locally or in the media), it should always be taken seriously.

Disruptions like excessive preoccupation with the body and self-cutting may be more common in girls, but boys also experience these disruptions.

If an adolescent shows a pattern of depression mixed with or alternating with a highly energetic, aggressive, or agitated mood, she may have a mood instability disorder. The most intense form of mood instability is called *bipolar disorder*, or manic-depressive illness. Bipolar disorder in adolescents may resemble this disorder in adults, and similar medications may help. Caution is warranted in labeling children with the specific term bipolar disorder or manic-depressive illness (see Chapter 2, **Mood swings**). The distinctions between various disorders of mood regulation (simple depression and mood instability) have implications for treatment (see Chapter 9).

Anxiety may show up in the form of panic attacks, ongoing states of generalized high anxiety, or excessive preoccupation about particular social situations. However, your adolescent's anxiety may not be so evident to you when she copes with it through avoiding what makes her anxious or when she distracts herself with rituals, compulsions, and preoccupations. These compulsions and preoccupations may focus on school work, particular sports, hobbies, or her body. At first it may be difficult to see that her excessive attention to school work or sports is a problem. However, upon closer examination, you may find that the excessive attention to studies helps your adolescent avoid other kinds of interests and activities that make her feel very anxious (see Chapter 1 for help on how to distinguish between normal variation and states that require evaluation or treatment).

The example below illustrates how one teen became depressed while coping with several major transitions, but gradually improved with family therapy.

Jennifer was an upbeat, engaging, and conscientious student. She had been a star on the school field hockey team and had many female friends. She found boys rather mysterious. She grew up in a family with just her mother, since her father had died when Jennifer was seven. Her mother had never remarried, although she had had a couple of long-term relationships with men.

At the start of the 12th grade, Jennifer seemed to have one positive experience after another. She began dating a boy, John, whom she had had a crush on from a distance. She was elected captain of her field hockey team and they were having an undefeated season. The coach at her college of choice told Jennifer that she was a shoo-in for acceptance.

About the time that her field hockey season ended, John broke up with her suddenly and began dating another girl, whom Jennifer never liked. Jennifer was devastated. She cried on and off about John and talked a lot about the end of her high school sports career, especially about missing the fun of practicing and playing with her friends. She complained she would never find such good friends at college. She began to express vague doubts about wanting to go to college. She moped around the house, showing no interest in joining her friends who called frequently. She let her school work slide and frequently got into arguments with her mother.

Her mother became more worried when Jennifer started making statements like "What difference does it make if I make friends in college? I'll only lose them too," and that life was basically just "disappointment and being alone." Jennifer's mother told her daughter that she thought she was depressed and needed to help herself. She suggested she make herself go with her friends, even if she didn't feel like it, as the isolation and inactivity only worsened her depression. She also suggested that Jennifer join the local YMCA to use the pool and exercise machines as she felt better when physically active. Jennifer agreed.

Her mother raised the possibility that she and Jennifer might see a therapist to iron out their differences, but mainly to talk about the big change that was coming in their life with Jennifer going to college. Jennifer agreed. Her mood began to improve pretty quickly as she engaged with her friends and got more physically active. The work with the therapist focused on Jennifer's worries about what it would be like for her mother if she were not around. She talked about remembering that her mother had gotten very sad for a long time following the death of Jennifer's dad. Jennifer's mother had had no idea that her daughter worried about her. Her mother in turn said that she had worried about how Jennifer would deal with boys in college and feared she would be hurt again. She worried that if that happened to Jennifer, she wouldn't be there to help her.

Both Jennifer and her mother were struggling through a major transition. It was particularly difficult because they had been so supportive of each other and so close after Jennifer's father died. As they talked in psychotherapy, they saw that their worries grew out of their care and love for each other and did not predict the future. Relieved of the burden of having to protect her mother, Jennifer seemed more positive about her college career. Her mother also became more supportive of Jennifer going to college, and she became more confident that Jennifer could cope with disappointments in relationships that might arise.

Disruption of relationships (attachment and sexual behavior)

The primary characteristic of puberty is the launching of the biological capability for human reproduction. This shows up in your adolescent's awakened interest in sexual matters and relationships. While the physical ability to have reproductive sexual intimacy with another person takes place, a competent combination of emotional, social, and physical abilities for ongoing sexual intimacy with another person takes many years to develop. The newly developed physical capability often must wait for the new combination of emotional and social abilities to catch up. This new combination has roots in earlier childhood when the ability to connect positively and sensitively with others is first developed.

Adolescents normally have a heightened involvement with peers and a heightened interest in sexuality (their own and others'). A teen's being either over-involved or under-involved with sexual matters may represent some kind of a problem, especially when sudden isolation and the absence of interest in others may also indicate the presence of some difficulty. For example:

- Withdrawal from peers and spending lots of time alone might point to a mood disorder, such as depression.

- Avoidance of peer contact and excessive concern about body image or sexual identity may be associated with a high level of anxiety.

- A decrease in social behavior may also be a defensive way of coping with the anxiety that accompanies the normal movement into more independence and freedom from parental oversight.

Over-involvement in social or sexual behavior can have various causes.

- Such behavior may be typical of your child's social circle: there may be lots of dating or partying. Your child may be comfortable with that or be overly social to try to fit in.

- Your child may be overly social or sexual to block out the emotional distress that is simply a part of adolescence.

- Your child may be trying to block out distress that may be particularly intense because it is part of a depression or a severe anxiety state.

- Your child may have overly sexualized behavior related to a past history of sexual abuse.

Experiencing feelings of sexual attraction for a same-sexed peer are neither voluntary nor indicative of a psychological disorder. Yet your adolescent may still experience great distress and strain because of such feelings. Since feelings of homosexual attraction may not be the custom of your family or your adolescent's peer group, your son or daughter may suffer great shame and isolation because of these feelings. The attraction may be brief and a small part of your adolescent's inner emotional life. Or it may be longer lasting and an important part of his or her sense of self. Talk with other parents whose son or daughter has gone through similar experiences. You might also find therapy of assistance in understanding your adolescent and your own responses to this unexpected situation (see Chapter 2, **Homosexuality**).

The story below illustrates how one adolescent girl and her mother negotiated some of the rough waters of adolescent sexuality.

> Allison had never been interested in boys until some time after her 15th birthday. Then she began to pay much more attention to her appearance, which had gone from gangly to voluptuous. The frequent telephone calls from her male classmates indicated that they had also noticed Allison's change.
>
> Her newfound popularity troubled her because her girlfriends seemed more jealous and envious than sympathetic to her confusion of how to deal with all the new male attention. She felt alone. She didn't know how to, or want to, talk with her mother about her thoughts about "hooking up" with one particular boy she liked and who seemed to like her.
>
> At a party where there was alcohol, Allison drank. She had to decide how far to go sexually. The boy she liked pushed the matter, and they had intercourse. The next day at school, Allison looked for the boy, with whom she believed she now had a special relationship. She was devastated when the boy ignored her. She became panicky when she learned a few days later that he was now seeing someone else. She began to wonder if she could be pregnant or could have contracted a sexually transmitted disease.
>
> Allison talked with a friend about her worries; the friend suggested she contact the local family planning agency. She did and was tested. She found out she was not pregnant and did not have any diseases, although she had to be retested in three to six months to be sure she wasn't infected with HIV. The counselor at the agency talked with Allison about sexual behavior and about birth control pills, and encouraged Allison to talk with her mother about the whole matter and return within the next couple of days to talk some more.
>
> Allison thought her mother would "kill me" if she learned that she had been sexually active. Yet she followed the counselor's advice. To Allison's surprise, her mother was more understanding than she had expected. Her mother went with her to the agency to discuss whether or not it made sense for Allison to start birth control pills, especially since she said she was never going to have sex again until she got married. While Allison's mother did not know if that would ultimately be true, she did know that her daughter needed her support. She also knew that her daughter needed as much information and guidance as possible.

Disruption of relationships (social custom)

Adolescents tend to be self-absorbed, largely as a response to the many physical and psychological changes they are going through. Yet they can also go through a time of heightened moral consciousness and tend to pay a great deal of attention to what is socially ethical and principled (especially in middle and late adolescence). Two of the many positive outgrowths of adolescents' remarkable intellectual and emotional development are their idealism and their constructive actions to make the world a better place.

Some adolescents remain more preoccupied with their own pleasures and fears than their more mature peers. Such immaturity may show up as short periods of behavior that seem antisocial. This does not necessarily indicate a serious disorder.

By contrast, ongoing patterns of lying, stealing, cheating, drug usage, or mistreating others or their property usually indicate that your child is having a very hard time managing ordinary adolescent emotional experience (like sadness, fear, anger, shame, or guilt). Failure to develop and maintain a solidly positive relationship with at least one adult may be part of the picture. Your adolescent may be unaware that his repetitive patterns of lying, stealing, etc. are driven by an attempt to avoid emotions like anger, shame, guilt, fear, or sadness. He may engage in antisocial behavior if he has no better way to manage and cope with those difficult emotions of adolescence. Signs that a teen needs professional intervention include:

- alcohol and drug usage that interferes with social activities, school performance, or relationships with others
- substance usage that has a compulsive/addictive quality
- behavior that results in legal difficulties (see Chapter 2, **Drug use**, **Stealing**, **Fighting**, etc.).

The example below illustrates how one young man's emotional struggles led him to begin taking drugs, which in turn increased his difficulties.

> Even before he ever got into trouble, Roger felt that he was the black sheep of his family. His older brother had been a star athlete and student in high school, and Roger knew that he had neither his brother's athletic ability nor his drive to excel in his studies. His parents had told him that he was just "as smart as your brother." But his grades never measured up and his parents were chronically disappointed.
>
> In school, Roger was drawn to a group of boys, who were not from his neighborhood, who seemed to accept him. When they offered to share their marijuana, he felt as if he now "belonged." Not long after that incident, he was using marijuana most weekends with his group. He then started using it at home on his back porch weekday evenings. Roger's grades, which had never been very high, took a dramatic turn for the worse. He lost his part-time job as dishwasher at a local restaurant because he was often late or did a careless job. He made different excuses for his problems, just as he made up stories about the pipes and other marijuana paraphernalia his parents found around the house. He progressively became more negative and oppositional at home.

When his older brother returned from college and realized what was happening, he confronted Roger. Their argument brought their parents into the matter. They arranged a meeting with a local substance abuse counselor a few days later. Roger held to the view that his marijuana use was not a problem. The counselor recommended a 12-step program for Roger but doubted it would go anywhere, as Roger was denying the problem and opposed to treatment. The counselor also suggested family therapy and recommended an evaluation to determine whether Roger had an underlying depression that needed treatment.

Roger's parents pursued these matters. They also considered a total change for their son. They began to inquire about alternative schools that he might attend as a day student. They even considered a residential school that specialized in helping boys with difficulties like Roger's.

Disruption of information processing (learning)

During adolescence gaining information about the world (both formally in school and informally in other settings) continues with increasing complexity. Examples include learning how to drive a car, how to negotiate money matters, and how to sift through information and pick out what's important on one's own. High school education leading towards college or technical/trade school becomes an important way station on the path to adult work, which in the modern world requires continued formal and informal learning.

If your adolescent has difficulties with learning and taking in the information appropriate to his age and career goals, this will affect his ability to succeed in the adult world. Interferences with learning must be tackled while your child is still in school, since unaddressed interferences with learning contribute a great deal to school dropout. And once out of school, your son or daughter will have many fewer services available for help.

Such influences include a specific learning disorder, handicapping attentional problems, or identifiable behavioral, cognitive, and emotional disorders. See "Disruption of information processing" in the section on school-aged children, earlier in this chapter, for more information.

Disruption of information processing (thinking)

Adolescence is a time of great intellectual development. Teens become better at thinking abstractly, and beyond their immediate sensory experience, than they were able during later childhood. They can wonder about the future and imaginatively manipulate ideas. They can consider other possibilities about a situation than what is immediately present and selflessly look at a situation through someone else's eyes. The human ability to give symbolic meaning to experience approaches full flower in adolescence.

Mental health professionals have identified a category of disrupted thinking, called a "thought disorder" or "cognitive disorder." This is in contrast to a mood or emotional disorder, discussed earlier under the disruption of emotional modulation.

A thought disorder, rare in younger children, is less rare in adolescents. If your teenager has a thought disorder, everything is to an extreme. Your adolescent may do or say things that don't make sense to most other people.

- What he says seems confusing. His behavior may seem odd, unexpected, or even dangerous.

- He may say things that seem overly concrete and simplistic or extremely abstract and difficult to follow.

- His speech and behavior may be extremely sped up or slowed down.

- Your adolescent may speak and act inappropriately perhaps with an extremely suspicious and overly guarded manner, or he may show no caution or careful judgment.

- He may see or hear things that others don't.

- These patterns of speech and behavior often represent a significant change from earlier ways.

This problem is not due to low intelligence or simple immaturity. Drugs or medical disorders may sometimes cause these changes. Seek prompt professional evaluation in such cases.

The example below illustrates how some teenagers can become overwhelmed with the multiple tasks they have to handle. In these cases, professional help is necessary.

Teddy's parents knew that their son was different from other boys the first time he went to school. The teachers reported that he liked to play more by himself, saying that he was building big castles to keep others out. He would often make up stories about his home and family that the teachers knew were not true. For example, he frequently spoke of a brother, even though the teachers knew he was an only child.

At home he was more engaging but never displayed much excitement or enthusiasm. He had many interests, although some were peculiar, like collecting dead spiders. Through his elementary years, the teachers noted that he continued to be a loner. He was hard to read emotionally: he had a blank look much of the time and he had odd responses to some of the classroom discussions. His parents tried to get him involved in after-school activities but he had no interest and invariably made such a fuss that they stopped encouraging him to go. He was never invited to other children's houses.

When puberty came, Teddy became irritable and hardly left his room. He even tried, unsuccessfully, to get his parents to let him eat his meals there. In the first year of high school, he developed a preoccupying crush on a girl, although he had never spoken with her. Despite his interest, he continued to dress rather carelessly and his personal hygiene remained poor. His father often had to remind him to shower.

He became obsessed with the girl and talked about her in front of his parents as if he had a relationship with her. He began telephoning her frequently and would hang up as soon as she answered. His parents found out about this because the girl's family had caller id and called his home to complain.

When his parents confronted him, telling him that this all was going on in his head and not in reality, he became angry and threatening. He accused them of not wanting him to be happy. Later that evening, they heard a thud and rushed to his room. They found him on the floor with a rope around his neck. He had tried to hang himself from the closet pole. Luckily, the pole had collapsed. Although he appeared physically okay, he was agitated and not making sense.

They brought him to the emergency room from which he was admitted to the psychiatric unit. It turned out that Teddy had been hearing voices for a few weeks. The doctors put him on medications and recommended that he enter an outpatient treatment program after the hospitalization. The program would give Teddy therapy, positive social experiences, and a chance to develop his abilities to relate better with his peers.

The movement into adolescence—with all the mental, physical, and social changes and tasks — was too much for Teddy's fragile mental state. He needed more time and support to help him with the complex passage through adolescence. He would get some of what he needed by participating in the therapeutic program and continuing to take his medications.

* * *

In this chapter, I have encouraged you to take a developmental perspective. We looked at particular normal tasks for your child or adolescent and then saw how symptoms related to a normal task. The developmental perspective is helpful in at least three ways.

- By looking at the normal and the particular symptom, you can more easily distinguish what is within the range of normal and what is problematic.

- You can figure out what is needed to move beyond the particular disruption/symptom.

- You can keep your whole child in mind: that part of your child having difficulties and that part of your child mastering the many tasks necessary to grow up.

The next chapter offers ten specific steps you can take that will help your child or adolescent get back on track, whatever kind of difficulty he or she might be having.

Chapter 4

TEN STEPS TO HELP YOUR CHILD GET BACK ON TRACK

Parenting is on-the-job training. This is particularly true when your usual way of helping your child with a problem doesn't seem to be enough. At those times, it is natural to become more uncertain and doubtful. You might begin to question the ways that you guided or interacted with your child and wonder about finding better ways to intervene to help her. Some of the steps offered in this chapter are probably things you have already been doing; seeing them here will encourage you to continue doing them. Other steps, or the perspective on the more familiar steps, may help you add something useful to what you are already doing. These steps can be helpful regardless of the type of problem your child is having and whether or not a professional is involved. These interventions will help you and your child be more psychologically available and better equipped for the task of getting back on track.

Organization of Chapter 4

The chapter is divided into ten sections, each discussing one of the following steps:

1. DO remind your child that you are both on the same side.
2. DO provide limits and reasonable expectations.
3. DO make sure your child has regular routines.
4. DO give your child encouragement.
5. DO help your child to confront fear.
6. DO NOT try to predict your child's future.
7. DO learn to see and appreciate small improvements and positive changes.
8. DO NOT let intense emotions dominate your interactions with your child.
9. DO remember that your child is not you.
10. DO take care of your own physical and emotional needs.

Each section gives the reasoning behind that particular step, some practical suggestions about implementing it, and occasionally some obstacles that you may encounter trying to carry out the step. At the end of each discussion I describe a situation that illustrates the ideas presented.

The steps

1. DO remind your child that you are both on the same side

Despite differences you and your child have in the present, ultimately you both want to help your child become a confident and capable adult.

Most children with troubling behavior or disturbed emotional states feel very alone. Your child may feel she is not understood or she cannot figure out how to make things better. This is even more the case if she senses that you are angry and disappointed.

Your child may also feel alienated and alone if she feels guilty. Children, and often adolescents, tend to see the world in simple black-and-white terms. Children often interpret difficulties that involve them as entirely their "fault." Your child may try to convince herself and others that the problem "is not my fault," while deep within feel that she is totally to blame.

If a child feels entirely at "fault," she may also believe that her parent is enormously disappointed and angry and that her parent's feelings might "never" change. This guilt and sense of alienation for "causing" the parent's emotional pain usually increases a child's anxiety, fear, and shame.

When strong, these emotions prevent good resolutions to emotional and behavioral problems and often increase such problems. Therefore, I encourage you to remind your child, and yourself, that you are both on the same side. Even if you feel disappointed, scared, or angry about the situation, remind your child that in spite of such feelings, you want to work together to make things better.

Fourteen-year-old Elizabeth and her parents frequently argued about many of her new interests: talking on the telephone to friends, sending "instant messages" instead of doing homework, and wanting to go to parties at the homes of people her parents did not know. Over the past year Elizabeth had become increasingly oppositional and defiant.

Although Elizabeth resisted when her parents held to limits, she did seem more responsive when they spent some time talking about how they were all trying to adjust to her getting older and desiring more freedom. In response to her parents' openness about their own struggles with her getting older, Elizabeth acknowledged more openly that she had been feeling torn between her wish to do things that were "fun" and feeling guilty about the distress her behavior caused her parents.

1. **On the same side**
2. Limits and expectations
3. Regular routines
4. Encouragements
5. Confronting fear
6. Predicting the future
7. Appreciating small improvements
8. Lessening intensity
9. Leading different lives
10. Taking care of yourself

Being on the same side helps you and your child find respectful solutions to your differences and makes your relationship stronger.

2. DO provide limits and reasonable expectations

Even those who have never been parents will offer the cliché: "children need limits." Many also know that children need reasonable expectations, like putting in good effort in school, behaving respectfully with others, doing family chores, etc.

However, it is not as well known that children usually do not thank parents for providing limits and reasonable expectations. Children in turmoil will often rebel intensely against unpleasant limits and strongly reject reasonable expectations. We know that children do better when there is predictable caretaking structure. A child becomes familiar with the experience of feeling safe when he confidently knows where he will go after school, when he will be picked up, and who will be there. The same holds true for the more uncomfortable limits and expectations, like how far he can go from home, who it is okay to be with, how late he can stay out, and what time he has to go to bed.

Despite your child's protests, setting boundaries for his safety and protection helps him feel cared about and worthy of care, and placing reasonable expectations upon him fosters a sense of fairness and confidence. All these experiences ultimately enable him to engage better with the unknowns in life.

So, what makes it so difficult to hold to these limits and expectations, particularly when your child's resistance to them is strong? The reasons range from cultural to emotional. Our society conveys the message that "you can have it all" and "the sky is the limit." That message doesn't acknowledge the sadness and disappointment that goes with experiencing a limit or a reasonable expectation. In addition, our society does not pay much attention to the difficulty of coping with the feelings of anger, shame, or sadness that we feel when we do not get something we want. In fact, often the simplistic message is that if you do not get what you want, or do not fulfill the expectations of others, then you are a "loser."

Ever since your child was small, you have had to confront and limit his "wants." Every parent has to develop a technique for dealing with the checkout counters which seem to be set up solely to entice a child. As your child grows, he wants more expensive things and is the target of more advertising. Your job of setting limits can become more and more time-consuming and challenging. How late can he stay out; where, when and how can he use the car; how are you to respond to finding out that he uses marijuana?

In fact, it may seem as though all you do as a parent is set limits on your child's or adolescent's persistent, persuasive, and occasionally intimidating, pursuit of what he wants. Your child may protest the expectations you place on him, expectations which you consider very reasonable: doing chores, being responsible about school work, or being kind to a younger sibling may lead to intense anger and resistance.

For some children, coping with the kinds of emotions raised by having limits and expectations—anger, shame, guilt, sadness—can be overwhelming. When handled poorly, these emotions contribute to a range of emotional and behavioral problems.

You may find yourself taking shortcuts in an attempt to keep your child from experiencing such painful feelings: you may pull back from having expectations, stop asking him to do the chores, put in good effort at school, etc. Your child's persistent requests, convincing explanations, angry protests, or sad withdrawals can wear you down. You may fear your child's response and feel like you are "walking on eggshells."

Contrary to your wiser tendencies, you may start giving in to your child's wants. A firm bedtime or driving curfew may get later. You may ask fewer of the questions that help you decide if you need to restrict who your adolescent spends time with, where he goes, or what he does. The setting up of limits can get more and more bewildering and you may feel like you have less and less influence or control. At such times, you may want to just let go of limits completely.

Acknowledge the desire, but don't do it! Remember, a parent's job is to set limits. A child's job is to protest about them, sometimes break them, and, as much as possible, bear the consequences of doing so. This back and forth struggle, done with as much respect, patience, and understanding as you can muster, is an important learning ground for your child. These exchanges are important opportunities for your child to learn to cope with the difficult emotions of sadness and disappointment, anger and fear, shame and guilt.

David was almost 15 years old. He had always followed his parents' rules and seemed to know intuitively how they wanted him to behave. However, over the preceding six months he had begun to change. He had let his hair grow longer than his parents thought acceptable. He persistently asked them to let him pierce his ear and frequently wanted to stay out much later than they thought suitable.

1. On the same side
2. **Limits and expectations**
3. Regular routines
4. Encouragements
5. Confronting fear
6. Predicting the future
7. Appreciating small improvements
8. Lessening intensity
9. Leading different lives
10. Taking care of yourself

They began to feel as if an alien had taken over their son. When they set limits, they were taken aback by his rageful outbursts. He complained bitterly to his grandparents that his parents deprived him of "all fun." When his grandparents asked more questions, David disclosed that he was talking about their prohibiting him from going to a rock concert that was 50 miles away from home and taking place on a school night.

The grandparents counseled David's parents to "hang in there." They knew, having raised three boys, that negotiating and tolerating limits would improve as David got older. They also knew that as David's parents gained experience, they would get better at managing limit setting and maintaining consequences when David broke the limits.

By continuing to hold to a structure of realistic limits and reasonable expectations, you are helping your child get back on track.

3. DO make sure your child has regular routines

Almost every parent would agree that a child should have regular routines for sleeping, eating, and exercise. A regular sleep routine means that your child has enough energy during the day to cope with the educational, emotional, and physical challenges that come up. A regular eating routine means that your child has enough nourishment, the important experience of being taken care of predictably, and an opportunity to enjoy food and conversation with the most important people in her life on a daily basis. A regular exercise routine means that your child is active each day, and her body thus is more likely to withstand injury and illness and to give her a sense of vitality.

Yet many parents, particularly parents of children with behavioral and emotional difficulties, often find it hard to establish and maintain regular patterns. Bedtimes are too late, sleep time too short, mealtimes erratic, and routine exercise spotty to non-existent.

Many factors contribute to this problem.

- Parents' days are hectic. Regular routines fall by the wayside even in their own lives.

- Our culture distracts from regular routines: television, computers, advertising, and fast food restaurants.

- School systems, pressured to "teach more," are cutting recess, when many children may have their only daily exercise.

- Sometimes fear, anger, and depression may disrupt your child's internal clock, resulting in erratic sleep patterns, disrupted appetite, and decreased energy levels.

What can you do to help your child get back on track to regular routines?

First, establish your own regular sleep patterns, eating times, and exercise periods. Your behavior is a powerful model for your child. Practice self-discipline by saying "no" to yourself and turning off the television, unplugging the computer, and establishing regular sleep and meal times. Do not watch television or use the computer before bed. This can show your child that you will do whatever is necessary to help her establish a bedtime routine. You will feel better during the day when you have had a good night's sleep and have some exercise. You will know the good feelings that come from looking forward to a regular mealtime and enjoying eating with your family. You also will learn how hard it is *not* to do something enticing and how difficult it is *to do* something not enticing. This will help you understand how hard it is for your child to hear your limits.

Second, make a written plan with your child and other family members that establishes regular routines. Acknowledge that changing the erratic schedule will not be easy, but that the goals are worthwhile in the long run. Consider establishing individual and family incentives for achieving those difficult goals. For example, some meals together might involve a special food. Your child might get to choose what the meal will be one day a week or help shop for and prepare the food. Or you might help your child exercise by getting her involved with organized activities like soccer teams, or play time with neighborhood children. Your participation, support, and encouragement help your child establish successful exercise patterns. You might say, "But that takes time!" Yes, it does, and it means that some other things don't happen. But you are demonstrating that you value this aspect of your life together and will sacrifice for it.

Third, practice. The particular schedules of eating, sleeping, and exercise will not become established until repeated for a while. You will need to reinforce and re-establish the routine when there is a lapse or disruption. Dealing with interferences is inevitable.

Sam, a nine-year-old boy, had attentional problems and trouble organizing and planning ahead. His appetite was erratic, particularly because he was on stimulant medication for his attentional problems. He often refused dinner and would eat later in the evening. He and his family gradually slipped into the routine of everyone else sitting down to dinner while Sam watched television alone. He had a hard time settling down to do homework and often watched television with his parents before he finished his work. He hated going to bed at a reasonable time and preferred to watch television until he fell asleep, often as late as 11:30 p.m. He preferred watching television to exercising.

1. On the same side
2. Limits and expectations
3. **Regular routines**
4. Encouragements
5. Confronting fear
6. Predicting the future
7. Appreciating small improvements
8. Lessening intensity
9. Leading different lives
10. Taking care of yourself

Sam's parents consulted with the pediatrician. She suggested that Sam join the family for dinner even if he didn't eat very much. She recommended his parents invite Sam to choose what foods were served and perhaps help cook one evening. They let him know that sitting down to dinner together is an important family ritual. The pediatrician also suggested that Sam get involved in some after-school physical activity; his parents could make this one of his "chores," for which he would get extra allowance. And she suggested that each evening Sam be required to do homework for an hour or read quietly if he did not have homework, and that the television be off for everyone during that time. Finally, she suggested removing the television from Sam's room if he could not turn it off at the appointed hour for bedtime. The doctor encouraged Sam to use a 15 or 20-minute relaxation tape to help him calm down before going to sleep.

While Sam protested about many of the changes, his parents discovered that with regular exercise he was more likely to have an appetite for dinner and to fall asleep at a reasonable time at night. Over time, Sam seemed to look forward to having meals together as a family. He particularly liked the evenings that he got to prepare dinner and receive praise from his family. Getting to sleep at a reasonable time also helped him have more energy in the morning and for school.

While the path to establishing eating, sleeping, and exercise routines may be difficult, you will find its impact on helping your child get back on track is worth the effort.

4. DO give your child encouragement

To parent well, just like to coach well, one must give many more positive encouraging comments than negative judgmental comments. Remember, your child's self-esteem is not fully developed and not self-sufficient. It needs nurturing and support to grow.

When your child is struggling to find effective ways to deal with his body, manage his emotions, cope with relationships, and take in information about the world, reality gives your child lots of negative feedback. He needs encouragement when encountering life's difficulties and praise when he overcomes those difficulties successfully.

My comments about encouragement and praise apply to all children (and to *any* intimate relationship). Encouragement and praise are especially important for children in emotional and behavioral turmoil; they often feel self-doubt and are sensitive to the negative opinions of family and friends.

As your child gets older, his mental life increasingly has a "mind of its own." He develops automatic ways to respond to difficult and painful situations. Some of those responses may not be in his overall best interest. However, they may be the best way he knows how to deal with a stressful situation. Encourage him as he struggles to find more effective ways to cope. Tell him what he's doing right. Doing so is more likely to affect positively his automatic ways of responding than criticism or belittlement.

You would never knowingly injure your child emotionally. But you, too, have automatic ways to respond to painful situations. Having a child with disturbed and disturbing behavior *is* painful. Do not over-use humor as a way to cope. A sense of humor can be a wonderful tool to help people handle difficult situations, particularly with adolescents. But what you may consider "just joking" or "only a little sarcasm or negative comparing" can deeply wound your child. Children with emotional and behavioral trouble often feel easily shamed, since they doubt themselves and are sensitive to the negative opinions of family and friends. Do not belittle your child with humor, sarcasm, or wounding comparisons. When discussing an issue that your child takes seriously, you may see the humor in it and try to make it a light discussion. If he seems to be getting agitated or angry, your son might feel belittled by your humor or teasing, even if you mean to be helpful. If you suspect that is the case, ask him how he feels about your humor at that moment. If indeed he does feel belittled, don't try to convince him to see the humor in the matter. Instead, acknowledge your misunderstanding and save your humor for later.

Jane, age 18, began struggling with depression and self-abusive behavior in January of her senior year in high school. She also began getting drunk at weekends. Any incident that she found emotionally distressing could trigger her to cut herself when she got home.

1. On the same side
2. Limits and expectations
3. Regular routines
4. **Encouragements**
5. Confronting fear
6. Predicting the future
7. Appreciating small improvements
8. Lessening intensity
9. Leading different lives
10. Taking care of yourself

Her mother was distressed and angry when she first learned of her daughter's behavior. However, she proposed supportively that Jane get into therapy as well as join AA. She encouraged Jane to get treatment and willingly drove Jane to therapy. She herself went to Alanon, the support group for family members of those with alcoholism. Jane reported that her mother's support and encouragement helped her change her behavior and deal with her emotional difficulties.

However, there was one lapse as Jane struggled with finding better ways to deal with her emotional distress than cutting herself. She told her mother that she had not been cutting for two weeks and wondered if she were pleased. Her mother shot back sarcastically, "Why should I be happy with something you shouldn't be doing in the first place?" Jane was angry and disappointed with her mother's response but didn't show it at the time. She secretly lapsed back into cutting herself on and off over the next two months.

Encouragement guides your child towards something positive that he can use for coping or feeling better. Sarcasm doesn't help him figure out what positive direction to go in; it simply points out what he's doing ineffectively, and often leaves him feeling shamed.

5. DO help your child to confront fear

Although we wish it were not so, our children's lives are filled with all kinds of distressing emotions. Most psychological and behavioral problems include difficulty coping with painful emotions. Children must learn to tolerate painful states and not feel overwhelmed by them. Confronting emotions means acknowledging an emotion's presence, understanding what triggered it, and not being compelled to act on it immediately. Confrontation is an important step in learning how to tolerate and cope with any painful emotional state. Since fear so often is an aspect of our emotionally troubling states, I have highlighted confronting fear as one of the ten basic interventions. But one can advocate for meeting almost any painful emotion—shame, guilt, sadness, or anger—head on.

Fear is sometimes called anxiety. Separation anxiety involves fear of being alone or abandoned. Social anxiety involves fear of being humiliated or shamed. Panic attacks often involve the fear of dying or losing control. Post-traumatic stress disorder involves the fear of being re-traumatized. Phobias involve the fear of a particular thing, place, or circumstance. Compulsive behavior involves the fear of consequences coming from not doing a particular action.

Help your child plan how to confront fear:

- **Exposure:** the first step in overcoming a fear often involves contact with the feared situation in a manner that feels reasonably safe to the person experiencing the fear. Finding a way for your child to feel "reasonably safe" may take time. Sometimes having a trusted friend or family member present may be enough to provide that feeling. Sometimes your child will need to approach the feared situation in small steps, such as first imagining the feared situation before being actually present at it.

- **Response prevention:** your child has to learn not to do what she usually does to avoid the feeling of fear. This requires your child not to flee a situation or not perform a compulsive ritual. This step is better carried out if your child feels "safe" enough to counter the rising feeling of fear.

- **Tolerance:** your child needs to learn to tolerate the feeling of fear, usually from 5 to 20 minutes, and experience that the fear begins to decrease. This step ultimately gives your child improved self-esteem, self-control, and confidence, and a sense of liberation.

Following these three steps helps your child learn that he can confront, tolerate, and overcome fear. Freed from having to act automatically on an upsurge of fear, your child can now choose a response that suits the particular situation. That choice likely will be based more on what is good or important to do rather than on simply trying to avoid fear.

This plan is clear and effective. But it is more complicated than it seems. It takes time and patience on the part of parents and child to work through the steps, because feeling safe or approaching the feared situation is usually done best in small steps.

Robert—an intelligent, sensitive, and thoughtful 15-year-old boy—had difficulty getting to school in the morning. His soft-hearted mother readily gave in to his feeble excuses as to why he could not go to school on any particular day. Yet she also understood that it was important for him to be in school and that some feeling of fear kept him from going.

1. On the same side
2. Limits and expectations
3. Regular routines
4. Encouragements
5. **Confronting fear**
6. Predicting the future
7. Appreciating small improvements
8. Lessening intensity
9. Leading different lives
10. Taking care of yourself

She decided to bring him to the mental health clinic. Once there, Robert spoke about feeling shame when he walked down the halls at the high school and a great deal of embarrassment when he was called upon in class and had to respond, even if he knew the answer to the teacher's question.

Robert was given medication that would decrease his feelings of shame and fear. He was told by his doctor that he would still have to confront his fear of attending school by going every day and confront his fear of shame by speaking up in class.

He wanted to overcome these fears. He worked with his therapist on listing his fears, starting with the small ones and working his way up to the big ones. It was important for him to feel in control of the process and that it wasn't moving too fast. His mother openly appreciated the courage it took for him to confront his fears.

Within two months, he was going to school regularly. Within three months he was frequently speaking up in class. He went off his medicine after five months. The therapist told Robert that he needed to keep "pushing the envelope" of his fear. He told Robert that some days he might feel his fear pushing back and restricting him, but he was to push back. He did this and discovered that on most days he felt no fear in those settings.

Confronting fear is done by tackling emotionally stressful situations and not avoiding them. This is the best way to decrease fear and keep it from blocking the path to useful or desired goals and positive self-esteem.

6. DO NOT try to predict your child's future

Don't be fooled into thinking that particular inherited traits, earlier life events, and old habits decide the future. When your child is struggling, it is natural to project those problems into the future and then imagine the unhappiness and suffering that "will" occur. But this just increases your agitation and worry in the present.

Humans' ability to anticipate is wonderful. We plan and carry out projects. We build buildings and cities, organize schools and armies, and write. But these complex undertakings rarely turn out exactly as planned. Unexpected events and circumstances interfere. There are unanticipated weather patterns, shortages of material, illness, competing needs, misunderstanding, etc. The more long-term or complex a project, the more likely things will not turn out as planned.

What could be more complex than the unfolding of a human life and the development of the human mind? We parents don't make our children into whom they become. We assist the process by working to meet day-to-day needs in a loving and attentive manner and by providing opportunities for our children to grow in particular ways.

No plan can guide an individual life or mind along a particular path. We cannot predict the future in general; we certainly cannot predict it about an individual life. Despite all the uncertainty, we still try to give our children's lives a shape and direction. We teach them how to plan and organize their lives. That is important. But that is different from predicting how things will turn out.

You are more likely to fall into the trap of thinking that you know how things will turn out when you are in pain and desperately want to know about the future. Realize that you are making the best decisions you can at the time. Later in life you may see things differently. Any time you make a decision, you cannot actually know the future.

Inherited traits influence the path your child takes. So do earlier life events and the behavior patterns that your child has developed. But no one can predict that path. We, our family members, and specialists all make predictions, occasionally with such certainty it seems we think we can see into the future. The best way to bring about a particular future is to act toward it in the present. Be open to learning new ways of seeing a situation. The opportunity for change and a new response is always possible in every situation that arises.

Matt was adopted at age three. He had been neglected and abused by his biological parents, who had a history of mental illness. Matt was tiny for his age and remained tiny. His adoptive parents gave Matt love, attention, and support.

Matt also had a learning disorder that was not identified until the third grade. He had trouble with organizing, planning, and keeping track of school-related tasks (like homework) and household chores. He also had a hard time reading social cues and making and keeping friends.

1. On the same side
2. Limits and expectations
3. Regular routines
4. Encouragements
5. Confronting fear
6. **Predicting the future**
7. Appreciating small improvements
8. Lessening intensity
9. Leading different lives
10. Taking care of yourself

His parents became discouraged. Knowing his early life history and family background, they imagined that their ten-year-old son would be handicapped with similar difficulties as an adolescent and adult. They imagined him disorganized, friendless, and even mentally ill like his biological parents. Despite their gloomy outlook, they kept giving him as many good experiences as possible. They also sought help from various therapists, doctors, and clinics.

Matt's difficulties at school worsened as the work load became heavier. At home, he would have angry outbursts that frightened his parents and him. His parents, in consultation with therapists and teachers, eventually placed him in a residential program paid for by his school system. He was in small classes with teachers skilled in special education; he lived in a group residence with other teenagers. He and his family received more intensive therapy than was possible as an outpatient. Teachers, residential staff, and the therapist worked with Matt on his social interactions with peers.

While in the program, from the age of 14 to 16, Matt grew a foot and a half. He began to use the many techniques others had given him to deal with his organizational and planning difficulties, as well as his emotions. He slowly learned how to get along with peers without alienating them.

His return to the regular high school was successful. He joined the ski team and, for the first time in his life, made friends on his own. It also became clear that Matt had musical talent. With only six months of guitar lessons, he was good enough to be invited to join an after-school band. Matt's parents were delighted with the changes that their son had undergone, but couldn't quite believe it. It took a while for them to fully let go of their "predictions."

Our history, biology, and old patterns each have a vote in influencing our response to some current event. Not one of them dictates the outcome. Focus on the present.

7. DO learn to see and appreciate small improvements and positive changes

Of course, you wish your child's problems were gone yesterday! As I discussed in Chapter 4, problematic emotional and behavioral patterns arise at different ages, and many of them diminish as your child matures. Just as it takes time to grow up, it takes time to heal or repair.

Continue doing all the good things you do to help your child. Noting small changes and improvements will help bolster your own hopefulness and your child's. Children have limited patience. One of your roles as a parent is to provide patience when your child hasn't developed enough. Do not focus too much on the long-term goal of where you wish your child were in terms of her problems. Doing so may keep you from seeing the small but genuine improvements and positive changes your child is making. Keep in mind that difficulties and problems are natural. Scars from the psychological wounds that we get in the process of growing up actually contribute to our unique strengths and interests as adults. Of course, those same scars contribute to our vulnerabilities and hindrances. By noticing your child's gains and positive changes, you increase the likelihood that one outcome of the difficulties is a psychologically stronger individual.

Sally's teenage daughter, Patricia, had been hospitalized for depression for four weeks. Sally wanted Patricia not to be depressed and to get back to school with a full academic load as soon as possible.

Sally couldn't understand why Patricia wanted an extra study hall, forgetting that her daughter needed time and tutoring to catch up on her work. Sally didn't realize that for Patricia, going to school, meeting her friends, and answering their questions after being out for four weeks was a big accomplishment.

Sally was jolted back to reality when she discovered that another girl who had been hospitalized at the same time as Patricia wound up back in the hospital just three weeks later. The stress of returning to school was just too much for the girl. Sally began to appreciate how much Patricia was accomplishing in the process of returning to her normal routine.

1. On the same side
2. Limits and expectations
3. Regular routines
4. Encouragements
5. Confronting fear
6. Predicting the future
7. **Appreciating small improvements**
8. Lessening intensity
9. Leading different lives
10. Taking care of yourself

Appreciating small improvements and positive change increases hope, supports patience, and helps your child get back on track.

8. DO NOT let intense emotions dominate your interactions with your child

It is normal to have an occasional strong emotional response to something that your child does or doesn't do, even if you later regret having been so emotional. For example, you might be furious that your depressed son is not doing his chores. Later, you may realize that you overreacted. Perhaps your anger was linked to seeing him depressed and feeling helpless to do anything about it. Or you may have felt terrified or panicked when your daughter didn't call home at the appointed hour. Later, you might realize that, in addition to the immediate situation, something else contributed to your fear, such as the fact that your own parents overreacted when you did not call home when you were your daughter's age.

Occasional overreactions happen. When you regain your balance, acknowledge to your child that you overreacted. This is not likely to undermine your authority. It will, however, help your child learn how to cope better when he overreacts.

Realizing when you are overreacting gives you insight into yourself and can help you not be so reactive to the momentary situation. Your intense emotional response may signal that something else, beyond the momentary situation, is in the "background" and contributing to your intense response.

If you often feel intense emotions in your relationship with your child, consider their impact on your child and your bond with him. Children often find intense emotions in a parent overwhelming. They often will miss the main message you are trying to send. For instance, your child may experience your mix of worry and irritation mainly as anger. Your child won't see your caring and may feel alone, unloved, and bad. Parents' anger is always hard for a child to tolerate. Your intense anger may push your child to erect a wall of "not caring" or to constantly be "walking on eggshells." Such reactions can further isolate a child who may already be feeling alone, unloved, and bad because of his difficulties. When you feel scared, anxious, or angry, wait until you are in a more settled state before discussing the issue with your child. Likewise, if your child is experiencing intense emotions, wait until he has settled down before entering into a discussion. It is better to help your child settle the overwhelming emotions of the moment than try to discuss rationally a highly charged topic.

If you are having frequent intense reactions, several steps may help:

- Talk with your spouse or child about their experience of your emotional intensity. This can give you a more objective view. Ask them to help identify when the intensity seems greatest. This will help you become more aware when it is happening. Try to sort out which emotions might be contributing most to your intensity. For example, your intense fear may be driving your anger. This means that you need to address your fear more than your anger. Express the emotion in words rather than actions. Use "I statements": say "I am feeling…" rather than "You are making me feel…"

- Give yourself ways to cope with the emotion in the present. See the emotion as coming primarily from within you, and give it time to pass.

- Do activities to distract yourself from the emotion of the moment, or try to bring up the opposite emotion. For example, count to ten (taking deep breaths with each number) to distract yourself from intense anger.

- If you feel intense shame, use humor, or look at yourself with compassion and acceptance.

John felt particularly irate with his daughter when she had angry outbursts after he had reprimanded her for not doing her chores. He could feel the steam building within his head.

| 1. On the same side |
| 2. Limits and expectations |
| 3. Regular routines |
| 4. Encouragements |
| 5. Confronting fear |
| 6. Predicting the future |
| 7. Appreciating small improvements |
| **8. Lessening intensity** |
| 9. Leading different lives |
| 10. Taking care of yourself |

He counted to ten and spent several minutes taking deep breaths before he could calm himself and talk with his daughter about her behavior. He knew that raging at her would not help her gain better control over her own angry outbursts. As he calmed down, he also realized that the intensity of her anger was probably linked to a sense of abandonment connected to her mother's unexpected death.

As he began to talk with her about how angry he felt in response to their situation, he realized that some of his own anger was also at his deceased wife. He felt that she had "caused" his feelings of abandonment by dying. He gradually realized that such feelings were natural, but caused him not to notice his true abilities and strengths. Indeed, he wasn't really a "helpless babe" or "incompetent jerk," as he felt when he didn't know what way to best help his daughter. Rather, he was a loving and caring father struggling with the hard work of making a life for himself and his daughter following the death of his wife.

However much you have to practice, decreasing the extent to which your intense emotions dominate your interactions with your child can help your child get back on track.

9. DO remember that your child is not you

You and your child lead different lives. On the surface, this statement seems self-evident. However, especially when emotions are a large part of our interactions with those we love, the distinctions become less easy to maintain. A joke captures the essence of this problem. Question: what is a sweater? Answer: something you put on your child when you are cold.

When your child was young, you had to rely upon your intuition, feelings, and past experience to figure out what your child needed. If you have a child whose temperament and likes/dislikes are similar to yours, you may not have had to confront the many ways that your child is different. But, if your child's way of experiencing the world is distinctly different from yours, you are continually reminded of the differences. With strong-willed children, this happens early. For others, the differences become evident as a child moves into adolescence.

Often the reminders of difference come abruptly. You may feel angry or disappointed when you expected that your child would respond in a way that doesn't happen. That expectation may be because you have blurred the distinction between how you *wish* your child to be and how your child *is*. Commonly, your wishes for your child have your own wishes for yourself mixed into them. For example, assume you would like to have your child learn to play the piano in order for her to experience the pride and pleasure in playing a musical instrument. Perhaps you wanted this as a child or actually did play the piano. Either way you wish to share in that pleasure with your child. This kind of mix is a normal part of intimate, loving relationships.

However, whenever a poor fit occurs between your wishes and your child's wishes, conflict can arise. Your side of the conflict may intensify when you find it hard to understand how your child could see the situation differently, or when you adamantly refuse to accept your child's different perspective and expect your child to see the situation like you do.

There is a constructive way to cope with the conflict. Hold to your own views and also fully appreciate that your child sees the situation quite differently. Feeling acknowledged even though opposed, your child is more likely to consider your views and reasonably listen to what you have to say, rather than emotionally rejecting what you have to say in order to maintain her identity or integrity. You are then more likely to respect the differences, communicate effectively about those differences, and successfully resolve them.

Your child is growing up in different circumstances than you did. You have been her parent; your own parent has not been her parent. Her sensitivities are not your sensitivities; your strengths are not her strengths.

Bill's son George was a smart, athletic, and energetic 16-year-old. Bill himself had been quite athletic in school and as a father had spent much time playing basketball with his son on their driveway court. Now that George was in high school and playing on the boys' basketball team, Bill proudly attended every game.

1. On the same side
2. Limits and expectations
3. Regular routines
4. Encouragements
5. Confronting fear
6. Predicting the future
7. Appreciating small improvements
8. Lessening intensity
9. **Leading different lives**
10. Taking care of yourself

George noticed during games that he would hear his father's voice calling out directions. At times his father's voice sounded almost as loud as his coach's. Occasionally George's team mates said that his dad seemed "really" into the game. On their drives home, Bill would critique his son's play. When George tried to object, Bill said he was "only" trying to get George to live up to his potential and accused him of being disrespectful.

George found himself having less interest in playing basketball, a sport he had formerly loved. He also felt mildly depressed. His lessened interest showed up as apathy on the court during a game. Seeing this, his father began criticizing George from the stands.

The coach, who had co-coached with Bill in a summer basketball league, saw what was happening. He had seen this before. Often a father would become so absorbed in his son's basketball accomplishments that he lost sight of the fact that he and his son might have different motivations and expectations. It was as if the father had stepped over some invisible boundary, hijacked a piece of his son's experience, and made it his own.

The coach spoke to Bill. He invited him to co-coach again in the summer basketball league and encouraged him to join a seniors' basketball league. He also told him that he was worried about George, who was taking basketball and himself too seriously. He wondered if Bill could help by talking with his son about "basketball not being everything." Bill said he understood. He became involved in his own basketball league and missed some of his son's basketball games because of his own games. George began having more interest in his own games and started swapping stories with his dad about their individual adventures in basketball. His mild depression lifted.

Strive to see your child's difficulties as belonging to your child, not to you. Then you will more likely see what your *child* truly needs to get back on track, rather than distortedly see what *you* might have needed to get back on track in similar circumstances.

10. DO take care of your own physical and emotional needs

Parenting is always hard work. You must plan for many practical matters. You must tolerate and absorb a wide range of emotional experience in order to help your child manage and learn to cope with his emotional life.

When your child is having problems, parenting becomes even harder. There are more unexpected practical issues and turbulent emotions to be dealt with. When your child is having difficulties, take care of your own emotional needs in order to avoid "burnout." Neglecting your own needs puts at risk your ability to be strong, thoughtful, and compassionate.

Burnout is physical or emotional exhaustion resulting from long-term stress. Physical symptoms might include headaches, poor sleep, weight gain or loss, backache, and digestive problems. Emotional symptoms might include increased anger and irritability, fatigue and apathy, increased anxiety and depression, and increased use of nicotine or alcohol/drugs. You can deal with burnout. One of your priorities must be to take care of yourself.

- Get enough sleep.
- Eat a good diet.
- Exercise regularly.
- Seek out activities and people that help you feel good about yourself.

- Make sure that you have a person who is a support for you and allows you to share your worry, frustration, and sadness about your child's difficulties. This person can non-judgmentally validate how painful your child's behavior or emotional states are for you and can remind you about what you are doing right for your child.

Keep a few perspectives in mind to help you more realistically cope with your situation and take better care of yourself.

- Parenting is not a job you can do perfectly.

- All parents have mixed feelings about their child at one time or another. You can feel sad and worried about your child's situation, guilty for the problem itself, and angry at your child because the problem exists.

- You alone did not create your child's problems; you alone cannot make them go away. If other family members tell you what you "should" be doing to "solve" your child's problems, let them know that such advice is not helpful and it's a complex situation.

- Your child's problems probably took time to come about and will take time to resolve. Set reasonable goals.

Conserve your strength and take care of yourself so you can be there for however long it takes to help your child get back on track.

Polly held a full-time job as a nurse, in addition to being a full-time wife and mother to three children. The oldest child, Alice, had recently been hospitalized for depression and had just returned to high school.

Polly was eager to support her daughter in her return to school. She did not want her daughter to get "stressed out" by school work, since she feared this contributed to her daughter's depression. She tried to be on top of Alice's homework requirements and know about all her assignments. She frequently contacted Alice's teachers to try to keep her daughter afloat.

1. On the same side
2. Limits and expectations
3. Regular routines
4. Encouragements
5. Confronting fear
6. Predicting the future
7. Appreciating the small improvements
8. Lessening intensity
9. Leading different lives
10. Taking care of yourself

Polly became distressed when she found out that Alice wasn't bringing home all her math homework. Wanting to support her daughter's faltering interest in math, Polly would take her own lunchtime to shop for any special supplies Alice said she needed to do math projects.

Polly was dismayed one day to find the supplies left at home in a corner of Alice's room on the day of the project. After hearing about this incident, Polly's husband said he thought that his wife was taking on too much responsibility for Alice's school work.

Polly spent time trying to fulfill her mothering responsibilities and work obligations, as well as to attend to Alice's school difficulties. She began to have less contact with her close friend Janet, with whom she used to jog four times a week. Their jogs were a wonderful opportunity to share emotional and practical struggles. Polly felt she couldn't spare the time since Alice's problems seemed so immediate. She found herself becoming increasingly irritated with her daughter. She stayed awake at night trying to think about what she was "missing." She tried to keep her worries out of her conversations with her own mother.

Polly became so anxious and depressed that she began to have difficulties at work. Ultimately, work problems led her to consult with a counselor in her company's Employee Assistance Program (EAP). He explained "parent burnout" to her and served as a sounding board for Polly's distressed emotions.

Polly began to realize that Alice's problems in school probably would best be helped by getting assistance from school staff. She spoke with the staff who agreed to track Alice's homework and provide any needed tutoring. Polly made an extra effort to jog with Janet at least two times each week. She slowly started being less irritable with her daughter. In fact, she became more available to hear of her daughter's difficulties in other aspects of her life, not just in school.

* * *

The ten steps described in this chapter certainly do not exhaust all the ways you can constructively help your child get back on track. For example, some additional ways to help your child include having regular organized play and leisure time with peers, spending frequent time together with family (nuclear and extended), doing work projects, community service, and just hanging out and having fun, or being part of some religious/spiritual community. Whatever those other ways may be, following these ten basic steps can provide a good foundation on which to build additional steps that would be more "customized" to the needs of your particular child.

The last step, taking care of yourself, naturally leads into the next chapter, which addresses your own emotional responses to having a child with difficulties. If you understand the feelings with which you are likely to struggle, you will be more aware of ways to take better care of yourself.

Chapter 5

COPING WITH YOUR FEELINGS WHEN YOUR CHILD SUFFERS

When my teenage daughter was unhappy and having difficulty with her peers, I mentioned my concerns to a friend. He listened to my anxious tone of voice and shared some of his own parenting worries. Then he sighed and said, "What my mother used to say is really true: you are only as happy as your least happy child."

When your child is unhappy—anxious, depressed, angry, confused, doing poorly in school, having trouble making friends—you share in that suffering. You share in it even though you may not feel it in the same way or with the same intensity. You find that you cannot sit by unemotionally while your cherished son or daughter is struggling. This is what keeps you awake at night thinking about your child's problem. This is what drives you to offer suggestions, make interventions, and speak with family or friends. Finally, this is what leads you to consider getting a professional consultation and treatment for your child.

Probably, over the past few months, you have tried many interventions on your own to help your child. But the problems and distress seem to persist. Perhaps you have talked with other family members or friends. Their suggestions might conflict with your understanding of your child, or their suggestions may not work. You may feel at your wits' end. While you may think that you are a poor parent and don't know how to intervene, it may be your own sense of disappointment, guilt, and worry about your child that is coloring your self-assessment.

Perhaps you recently learned of your child's difficulties and feel quite confused and paralyzed about what to do or how to think about the problems. Or you may have had some ongoing sense that your child is a little off-track. Although your distress may be at a low level, it has motivated you to seek help. By whatever route you got there, your emotional equilibrium has been disrupted and you're looking for ways to get you and your child back on track.

You may have heard the expression that every problem is actually two problems. One problem is *practical*: you can address this by getting more information and facts to help you figure out what to do. The other problem is *emotional*. This is addressed through tolerance, compassion, and wise management.

Most of this book addresses the practical problem of how to respond effectively to your child's emotional and behavioral difficulties. In this chapter, I directly address the emotional part of the problem of having a child with difficulties: your experience as a worried, distressed parent. The feelings discussed below are normal when someone you love is suffering and your enjoyment of life is at a low point. You might be flooded with different painful feelings all at once, or you may pass through stages that are dominated by one feeling or another. Of course, as a parent, you may experience such feelings whatever the age of your son or daughter: from toddler through adult. Understanding more about these feelings may help you cope better with them, and how you handle your feelings can impact on how your child deals with his/her struggles.

Organization of Chapter 5

I first address the emotions of guilt, shame, fear, anger, and sadness. After describing each emotion—how it may be experienced, how it can be a hindrance, and what may help you cope with it—I give a clinical example. In many of these little examples, I follow one parent of a teenager as she experiences the various emotions in response to her child's suffering.

I then talk about coping with the pain caused by not being able to fulfill all your expectations of protecting and caring for your child. This includes the proposal of a "Parents' serenity prayer."

Your own painful emotions

Guilt

Parental guilt seems to surface in two forms. One form arises when a conscientious parent feels excessively responsible for a child's difficulties. The circumstances that can trigger this intense feeling of responsibility might include a divorce, your own medical illness, or a family history of mental disorder.

Guilt keeps you from seeing that your child's particular difficulties have many contributing causes. You may irrationally lay total responsibility for your child's difficulties at your own feet. Intense guilt, or self-blame, may lead you to say or do things that make the situation worse. Your guilt may be so strong that you cannot recognize or appreciate all you have done to help your child.

Cindy's 15-year-old daughter Margo had been having many difficulties over the past several months. Margo had been caught skipping school several times, and violated her curfew regularly. When at home, she mostly kept to herself in her room; she often stayed up late sending emails to her friends. The guidance counselor at school expressed concerns about Margo. She told Cindy that two other students had told her that Margo had said she was depressed. The students feared that Margo would hurt herself.

Cindy's husband Frank had left the marriage about a year earlier. He had only sporadic contact with his daughter. Cindy worked full-time. When Cindy first heard about Margo's difficulties, her first response was to feel that the guidance counselor was saying that she was a "bad mother." She felt she had "totally" failed her daughter. She felt tremendously guilty, which came out largely as feeling very angry with herself. As a result, she yelled angrily at Margo when she next saw her, "Why didn't you tell me you were depressed?" Margo did not hear the guilt and concern in her mother's angry voice; she only heard the anger. She then felt guilty herself.

A second, less obvious form of guilt conceals the personal sense of responsibility. In this case, you do not direct your criticism and excessive responsibility at yourself. Instead, you redirect your harsh judgments and blame for your child's difficulties toward someone else: your partner, your other children, your troubled child, teachers, etc. You may find it hard to consider that your interactions with your child may be a factor in your child's troubles. Obviously, this form of managing guilt also keeps you from seeing your child's difficulties as complex, with many causes.

It can be even harder to cope constructively with your guilt if your well-meaning but misguided family members or neighbors blame you.

Cindy was angry with her husband, who had emotionally abandoned his wife and daughter. He was depressed and withdrawn. He was drinking heavily at weekends, and barely maintaining a regular work schedule. Underneath her anger, Cindy felt guilty that she had "caused" her husband to become depressed and start drinking.

Cindy talked with her mother about the situation. She wound up feeling even further demeaned and misunderstood when she heard her mother's view that the marital situation and Margo's difficulties were Cindy's "fault." Only much later in the course of dealing with her daughter's problems did Cindy come to see that her mother's view was wrong and that she didn't have to accept everything her mother said as true simply because her mother said it.

Your guilt, however you experience or deal with it, comes from a deep sense of sadness and helplessness about your child's difficulties. Your guilt may decrease when you realize that professionals do not blame you and that many different factors contribute to your child's problems. Your guilt may decrease even more when you see your child respond to helpful treatments.

Shame

You may also feel shame about your child's difficulties. You can feel particularly ashamed when your child has difficulties even though you try to make things better. It is natural to want your child not to have emotional and behavioral difficulties. Even though you know that difficulties are a part of life, you may view the very presence of a problem in your child as your own shameful defect or impairment. Often, the more you experience your child as a part of you, and as overly identified with you, the more shame you may feel when difficulties arise (see Chapter 4, Step 9: DO remember that your child is not you). This feeling may be made worse if other parents, and other parents' children, do not seem to be having emotional and behavioral problems. If we don't see their struggles, which often happens, we can feel alone and like a failure as a parent. Intense shame can keep you from seeking treatment or interfere with the treatment process itself.

> In addition to feeling quite guilty about what had happened to her daughter, Cindy also experienced great shame. She had waited over two weeks to tell her brother about the situation, even though she knew he would be quite supportive of her. When she first accompanied her daughter to the mental health clinic, she kept her head down when any person came into the waiting room, fearing she would be identified. One source of the fear was her dread of how humiliated she would feel if a co-worker or neighbor entered the room.
>
> Cindy joined the mother–daughter weekly therapy group sessions that were part of the treatment plan. She heard about others' difficulties and began to feel more like a mother struggling with a depressed daughter and a difficult situation and less like a failure as a parent. She was nervous when her daughter began to speak up in the group. But she was moved when she heard her daughter express her own anguish, disappointment, shame, and guilt at her parents' marital difficulties. She was also touched when she heard her daughter talk with kindness and understanding to other girls in the group who were struggling with depression. Cindy felt compassion towards her daughter and herself. She also felt relief as she saw Margo's mood and behavior begin to improve.

The intensity of shame, and the connected urge to hide, is lessened by compassion, which occurs when there is an awareness that a difficult and painful situation calls for some tenderness. Compassion will reduce shame regardless of the situation that triggered it. Shame-diminishing compassion may come from within you or from others. It will come from within when you understand that parenting involves a lot of "on-the-job training" and that you are not the only one who at times feels like a failure.

Fear

Parents inevitably feel scared and worried when they feel helpless to affect a child's emotional and behavioral troubles. You may irrationally expect the worst and project your intense worry and fear into the future and imagine very painful scenes for yourself and your child. Without realizing it, you may come to believe that your worries *are* the future! This can happen, even though rationally you know that no one can know the future. Such fear responses increase when you keep your worries to yourself. If your worries are quite strong, you may actually feel despair.

> Cindy spoke in the group of how frightened she had felt when she first became aware of her daughter's struggles. She had a younger sister who had attempted suicide at about Margo's age and had many years of untreated depression and substance abuse. Cindy knew in her mind that Margo, who had no substance abuse problem, was different from her sister. Despite this understanding, Cindy shared that she had had frequent worries that Margo would "turn out" just like her sister.

You can reduce the intensity of your fear and worry by doing one or all of the following:

- talk with a professional
- learn more about your child's problem
- discover that there can be helpful interventions.

Anger

The same unwanted situation that triggers guilt, shame, and fear can also trigger anger. You want the difficulties for you and your child to disappear. Any reminder of them can trigger your anger, which inevitably comes up when you feel helpless, alone, and overstressed. Anger also may come up in response to your fear and guilt that was triggered by your child behaving or feeling a particular way. Similarly, you may feel guilty when you realize that anger directed at your child is usually not helpful and probably worsens his already overwhelming feelings.

Keep in mind that angry feelings are normal. Anger can energize us to address a problem and to take conducive action. Yet intense anger can lead to hurtful angry words and angry behavior which, if directed at your child, may intensify your sense of guilt, shame, and worry. Angry speech and actions are much easier to control than angry feelings. Generally speaking, it is good to control angry behavior. However, because you have little control over whether an angry feeling comes up within you, acknowledging and accepting the presence of such a feeling may be the most immediately helpful response you can have. More often than not, especially if not acted upon, the feelings of anger at your child diminish and pass, and the likelihood of injurious angry behavior decreases. At that point the energy of your anger may be used to say and do something more constructive to address the situation.

> Before entering the support group, Cindy was primarily aware of her anger. She felt angry with her husband for leaving and having minimal contact with Margo and herself; she felt angry with Margo for having difficulties and not telling her. She felt angry with herself for not seeing her daughter's difficulties before the school counselor told her.

> As she progressed with the group, and her own individual therapy, she came to see other feelings in her that she had only felt as anger. As she began to see more of her complex emotional response, the intensity of her anger lessened.

The passing of anger occurs with time. You can help it pass by remembering to appreciate your child's experience and perspective. Hold on to the understanding that your child is having a painfully difficult time and that the hurt and anger you are feeling was not intended by your child. Remember that your life has its own stress that can lead you to feel helpless and alone, independent of your child's difficulties. If you're in such a place and discover that your child is having a problem, you might respond with anger at being further burdened.

Since anger often decreases and fades away when you do not feel so alone with your struggles, it can help to talk about the problem with someone: a spouse, family member, friend, or professional. Likewise, the sense of helpless anger may decrease when you see that you can take positive action and helpful steps that make the situation better.

Sadness

Guilt, shame, fear and anger that he or she may incorrectly come to believe may precede or accompany feelings of sadness. When not acknowledged or managed well, these other strong feelings can move us away from more realistically accepting and addressing a difficult situation. In contrast, sadness often signals some degree of acknowledgment and acceptance of a painful and unwanted reality.

Sadness is normal. It commonly arises when you fully grasp that your child is going through a very difficult time and that you have limited ability to keep it from happening. Acceptance is not simple resignation. In fact acceptance, which often takes some time to reach, may let you see beyond the current situation and imagine new options. It allows a place for the hope that things can be improved.

Sometimes, however, sadness may come too soon and too strong—more like hopelessness and despair than acceptance. A person may *feel* so overwhelmed with guilt, shame, fear, or anger that she may incorrectly come to believe that the situation itself is overwhelming and feel despairingly sad. As with all emotions, time plays an important part in the passing of sadness. While sadness cannot be rushed, its pain can be softened by self-compassion—tender understanding for yourself and what you are experiencing.

> While Cindy commonly welled up with tears when she was angry and frustrated, she felt limited relief at those times. However, as she faced her own guilt and shame, she began to feel sadness for what she and her daughter had had to experience. The sadness that accompanied her tears had a quality of acceptance and relief. After many episodes of sadness, Cindy began to feel a sense of hope

for herself and for her daughter. Instead of feeling overwhelmed most of the time, she began to feel that she and her daughter were capable of confronting and managing the emotional and practical difficulties in their lives.

It's probably no surprise that the complex emotional responses you undergo do not simply disappear when you seek professional help. In fact, your feelings might get stronger at the start of treatment. Despite society's progress in lessening the stigma associated with seeking professional mental health treatment, it still exists. Like Cindy, you may feel inadequate or like a failure as a parent if you decide to seek professional help.

Some of these feelings grow out of the sadness and disappointment you may feel for not having protected your child from life's troubles. Though rationally you may grasp that growing up is difficult and getting off-track is very human, emotionally you may not be so understanding and compassionate. You may agree, rationally, that parenting is complex and difficult. Yet emotionally, you may feel like a failure for not having found the "right" intervention for your child.

Unfortunately, our society's emphasis on independence and "doing it yourself" encourages such feelings. You may hear subtle, or not-so-subtle, belittling comments from family members or friends because you have decided to seek professional help.

You may have to struggle not to let your fear of being seen as a failure guide your behavior. Like Cindy, you might find yourself not telling some family members that you are seeking help for your child. You may do this even though they are aware of the difficulties.

In the past, some people have mistakenly viewed the parents' feelings of failure and inadequacy—which come up in *response* to a child's problems—as the *cause* of the child's problems. For example, consider the changes over the past 45 years in our understanding of a severe behavioral and emotional disorder of childhood: autism. Professionals once thought that the reason a child with autism had difficulty forming an attachment with his/her mother was mainly due to the aloof quality in the mother.

Professionals now know that view was wrong. We now understand that parental behavior that was seen as a "cause" of the child's disorder is more accurately viewed as a *reaction* to the profoundly disturbing experience of having an infant or toddler who does not react positively to maternal nurturing. Later, observers found that parents responded in many different ways to autistic children, sometimes more constructively and sometimes less constructively, depending upon their understanding of the problem, practical means for coping with it, and resources for managing their own emotional distress. Autism is now known to be a severe developmental disorder present from birth. But many parents suffered emotionally from the wrong view about the cause of autism. As those parents learned that autism was a biological disorder and not caused by them, they felt less guilty and more angry at the medical establishment.

Parents of autistic children must still make peace with feelings of guilt, shame, fear, anger, and sadness, as must all parents who have a child with other kinds of emotional and behavioral difficulties. This task is easier when the larger community acknowledges the reality of childhood mental illness, doesn't stigmatize it, and supports proper treatment for it. The stigma about treatment for mental health problems is more likely to fade away when our society recognizes more deeply just how demanding and difficult parenting can be.

Parents' serenity prayer

You know that parenting is hard work. Even when times are joyful, thought and effort are always required. More often than you wish, life with your child doesn't go as smoothly as you had planned. Yes, parenting is hard work and often feels like on-the-job training. While this is particularly true for a first-time parent, it is true as well for the experienced parent. Each child is a new experience—with a different temperament, different experience, and different position in the family—even if the gender is the same.

You will truly feel that parenting is on-the-job training when your child has some unforeseen difficulty and you are trying to figure out how to help. Fortunately, as long as you are a parent, you can get better at the job of helping your child learn to cope with life effectively.

However, many times your knowledge, skills, and loving relationship are severely taxed by your child's difficulties. The loving bond with your child keeps you going forward. But you can feel very challenged, even overwhelmed, by having to choose between so many possible responses to any one situation. At those times, you may feel that your emotional equilibrium is about to crumble and that you are at the limit of your ability to help or even "keep it together." You realize that you have limits in your ability to care for, protect, and help your child. You might feel that the best that you can do is to avoid making matters worse for your child or yourself.

These can be painful and humbling times in your parenting journey. Surprisingly, these may also be the times when you grow the most, particularly in your ability to distinguish between what you can and cannot do for your child. The need to make this distinction increases as your child gets older and you are less able to direct your child's life path. You must constantly adjust to the reality of your child changing and cope with the emotions that go with facing these changes.

The bad news is that the wisdom to distinguish between what you do and do not have control over in your child develops painfully slowly. The good news is that you can continue to gain wisdom throughout your journey as a parent.

When you feel challenged in the ways I've described, draw upon the parents' "serenity prayer," a variant of the serenity prayer used in 12-step programs. It asks for three things:

1. the serenity to accept those things in my child I cannot change
2. the courage to help change those things that I can
3. the wisdom to know the difference.

To *accept those things in my child I cannot change* means being aware of and acknowledging reality: at this point in time, even with whatever help you can offer, your child is not able to be the person you wish him or her to be. Your expectations may be reasonable and loving; they are your wishes for your child. Yet your wishes are not your child. Nor are your wishes being fulfilled by who your child is right now. Acceptance is not just passive tolerance of an unwanted situation. Acceptance helps you actively validate and acknowledge who your child is and what your child is struggling with.

Deep within the prayer is also the acceptance of your own limits as a human being and a parent. Having limits does not mean you are a bad parent; it means that you, like all parents, are imperfect. The prayer begins with a request for *serenity*, or the capacity for self-compassion and kindness towards yourself. It is necessary because, as you become more accepting, you may also have to give up a piece of a dream about your child, and perhaps about yourself.

> Ralph was an attractive, bright, eight-year-old boy who was shy and subdued. His outgoing father was continually encouraging Ralph to be like his cousin, Stephen, an outgoing athletic boy the same age. The more Ralph's father pushed him to participate in more robust activities with others, the more Ralph withdrew. Not only did he resist playing soccer, but he withdrew from his beloved chess club.
>
> Ralph's father sought professional consultation because of his son's withdrawal. Through working with his son's therapist, he began to accept his son's sensitivity to social pressure. He also worked to accept his own limits as a parent and that he wasn't a failure just because he couldn't "fix" his son. Ralph's father was surprised to find that his son became less withdrawn as he became more accepting of his son and his shyness.

Asking for the *courage to help change those things that I can* implies a desire for patience, understanding, and determination, which are necessary for bringing about change in your child, particularly if your child's fear, willfulness, or limited abilities make change difficult. Courage will help you through your own feelings of doubt, hopelessness, and frustration that are often part of trying to bring about difficult change.

To have *the wisdom to know the difference* requires good judgment to know when to let go and when to push, argue, and try to influence. It is expressed in the familiar recommendation to "pick your battles." This wisdom develops over time, through your own successful and unsuccessful experiences, what you learn from others, and your own thoughtful reflection and consideration.

As Ralph's father became more understanding and accepting of his son's shyness, he also began to support his son's interests, even though they were not his own choices. He set aside extra time to listen to his son passionately talk about various chess strategies, and took his son to local tournaments. This was difficult at first, since Ralph's father had a different temperament and was drawn to more outdoor, robust physical activities. Instead of focusing on what his son wasn't interested in, he focused on what his son was experiencing and achieving: his enthusiasm and increasing competence and success in tournaments.

If you do seek professional help, you may find that this, too, involves deciding when to let go of expectations and when to hold onto them. You will need to find a balance between the pull of the hope that you will help your child on your own and the pull towards accepting outside help. Asking the following questions may help.

- "What kind of relief, through my loving relationship and thoughtful presence, can only I offer to my child?"
- "What kind of relief, through psychotherapy and/or medication, can only a professional offer to my child?"

This addition to the Parents' serenity prayer may help in such a situation: "Grant me the wisdom to find a sensible balance between what the professional has to offer my child and what I have to offer my child."

The next section of the book covers topics that come up if you seek professional help for your son or daughter. Chapters 6–11 will help as you try to find that sensible balance between what the professional has to offer your child and what you have to offer.

Section II

PROFESSIONALS' INTERVENTIONS

These next six chapters address topics that come up as you try to get your child professional help. Once you have decided to consult a specialist (for evaluation or treatment) you have new information to deal with and new decisions to make. These chapters offer practical information, but also contain the names of various treatments, professionals, medications, etc. that may be new to you. With so much new to deal with as you seek proper mental health treatment for your child, you may feel like you are lost in a confusing and frustrating maze. I hope the following information will help you navigate that maze and see it more positively as a path towards helping your child get back on track.

Before the first chapter on professional help, I present a brief overview of how the child mental health system has evolved over recent years. This will help you better understand how today's system works. I focus particularly on child psychiatric practice, including my opinion about the current emphasis on the biological/ pharmacological perspective for making sense of and treating children's difficulties.

Changes in child mental health treatment in recent years

The practice of child mental health treatment has changed dramatically since 1975. When I trained (1974–76) and began working at private and public non-profit clinics for children and families, the child psychiatrist would provide a range of treatments. This usually involved doing individual play therapy with the child, seeing the parents in ongoing consultation or family therapy, and prescribing medication.

Very few medications were used with children in 1974. Children were rarely diagnosed as "depressed," and only one main category of medication could be used to treat depression. Antidepressant medication almost always was used only with adults. Except for Ritalin, there were few medications for other kinds of problems.

Children were treated primarily with just psychotherapy. Many children benefited, but others improved only slightly or could not take advantage of what was offered because their symptoms were so disruptive. Many very non-responsive children needed hospital treatment.

By the mid-1980s, different kinds of medication became available. Children who had not responded well to just psychotherapy began to receive medication. Clearly, for some children, receiving both therapy and medication increased their chances of improving. For children with very intense and disruptive symptoms, medication meant that they could be taken care of as outpatients, rather than being hospitalized or having to go into residential treatment programs.

As more helpful medications became available, child psychiatric practice changed. Whereas in the past the psychiatrist provided mostly psychotherapy, nowadays a child psychiatrist spends time mostly doing medication consultations and providing medication treatment. Consultations usually happen when a non-medically trained mental health colleague raises the question of whether medication might help. That colleague (a social worker or psychologist) is usually the one who now provides ongoing psychotherapy for a child.

This split arrangement (one person doing psychotherapy and one providing medication) means more children can receive proper treatment. It developed for two reasons:

1. There are not enough child psychiatrists to provide medication treatment and psychotherapy for those children who could benefit from both.

2. There are more social workers and psychologists available for treating children with psychotherapy than there were in the past.

Child psychiatrists spend more time prescribing than they used to, so medication is more available as a part of treatment. In addition, there are now more different kinds of medications from which to choose: for any specific symptom, there are typically two or more medications available for treatment. The same medications used to treat adults are used to treat children, although medication treatment for children begins at much lower doses and the dosage is increased more slowly. Another change from the past treatment is that there are certain types of psychotherapy once used only for adults (such as cognitive behavioral therapy and dialectical behavioral therapy) that now are being used with children and adolescents. There is also more research support for the effectiveness of different kinds of psychotherapy.

For many children, the "explosion" in the use of medication has been valuable. Children who might have been frequently sent out of class for misbehavior (caused by excessive distractibility and problems with attention) now take medication and spend more time in class learning. Children too fearful or too depressed to go to school now attend. The self-esteem of a child who goes to school or is able to stay in class is higher than one who can't make it to school or gets thrown out of class often. A child with improved self-esteem more likely will listen to adults. When that happens, home life goes more smoothly and getting ready for school and other transitions is easier for everyone. Less conflict usually leads to better relationships and even more positive self-esteem.

However, despite these major benefits of medication, I believe that caution is necessary. For some children, medication that held the promise of being helpful may, due to allergy or serious side effects, turn out to be harmful. There have been recent stories in the newspapers of children who may have been seriously, even fatally, harmed by medication. Worried parents understandably find it intimidating to approve of their child being on psychiatric medication.

- We do not know enough about medication's short-term effects on children.
- Children are still growing and may be sensitive to long-term effects of medication.
- Human problems come about for many complex reasons, many not properly treated by medication.

Most child psychiatrists share in this caution. They decide to use a medication after a careful assessment of the needs of a particular child. They base their decisions about a particular medication's benefits and disadvantages on their professional experience, discussions with colleagues, and reports by researchers in professional journals.

But some reasonable points of view go against this perspective of caution. Parents naturally want to find quick relief for their child's distress. Medication has shown that it can lead to dramatic improvement. When it works, medication can seem almost miraculous. And there are also some less sensible points of view that go against this perspective of caution:

- Many naively believe that complex medical and psychological problems can be adequately addressed just by taking a pill.
- Many naively believe that a symptom might be viewed only as a nuisance, to be gotten rid of, rather than a potential warning sign that some important but as yet unseen problem needs attention.
- Many hold the narrow and shortsighted economic view that favors change through the use of a fairly inexpensive pill alone over change that also involves more expensive psychotherapy.

Most experienced child mental health specialists doubt such simplistic views because they know that behavioral and emotional problems can have multiple and complex causes. They know that psychotherapy is helpful in treating such problems. And most recommend that children use medication in combination with some form of psychotherapy, not on its own. Nevertheless, there is growing pressure on child mental health professionals to treat children in a short period of time with medication alone. Pressure comes from:

- stressed parents who want their child to be symptom-free quickly

- insurance companies (public and private) that want treatment to be brief and economical
- pharmaceutical companies that bombard physicians with persuasive information about the newest drugs.

Parents and professionals must be sure not to shortchange the very children they want to help. When parents phone and ask for "just a medication consultation," I try to offer an alternative to the view that sees a child's disorder as purely a "chemical imbalance." Section II of this book is based on the view that when thinking about the best treatment for a child, both psychological and biological (pharmacological) perspectives should be included.

Chapter 6

EVALUATION AND TESTING: WHY, WHAT, WHO, AND WHERE?

My goal in this chapter is to give you enough information to make your experience with psychological testing less mysterious and less anxiety-provoking. I want you to know enough to be able to explain the process to your child. I also provide information about other kinds of evaluations, done by child psychiatrists and pediatric neurologists, for these same goals.

I use the term "evaluation" to refer to the general process of assessment, which means looking more closely at a problem. I use the terms "test," "tests," or "testing materials" for the specific tools or materials used during an evaluation (particularly by a clinical psychologist).

The complex process of evaluating and testing children who have emotional, behavioral, and learning difficulties can be confusing. A school counselor or social service worker may have told you to call a child psychiatrist and get a psychological evaluation for your child. But a child psychiatrist does not do psychological testing. A psychological evaluation is a complex procedure that mostly involves paper and pencil testing and is given by, or under the direction of, a clinical psychologist. A child psychiatrist relies on the test results to help guide treatment.

If you phoned a professional requesting a "psychological evaluation," you might be asked, "Why was psychological testing requested for your child?"

- You might say that your child is having some emotional and behavioral difficulties, or that there is concern about your child's progress in school.

- You might say that no one has told *you* why your child should be tested. You then might need to go back and talk to the individual who suggested that you get the evaluation.

- You might say that your child had some testing by a school psychologist, who then recommended additional, more comprehensive evaluations by a neuropsychologist.

Such complexity, confusion, and miscommunication regarding psychological testing is common.

Organization of Chapter 6

This chapter has four main sections:

1. **"Why"**: this consists of the reason your child might be referred to a particular child mental health specialist for evaluation and testing, what might be learned from such tests, and how that information might help your child. For example, the school personnel notice your child isn't learning as expected; tests show that she has a learning disorder, and specific interventions are recommended. Or your child's therapist says your child isn't responding as expected, testing shows that he is more depressed than appeared, and the focus of work changes or a referral for medication evaluation is made.

2. **"What"**: this includes what tests are used and what each assesses. I outline five main types of psychological and neuropsychological testing, and also mention different types of non-psychological testing.

3. **"Who"**: this focuses on which specialist does the testing. I distinguish between a confusing cadre of health care professionals, including pediatricians, neurologists, child psychiatrists, psychologists, physical therapists, occupational therapists (see also Chapter 7, *Questions about Treatment: Who Are the Helpers and Where Are They?*).

4. **"Where"**: this includes where you might take your child for an evaluation.

The chapter ends with a brief example to illustrate how some of the psychological tests are used.

Why was the evaluation or testing requested?

All of the adults involved with your child may realize that he is having difficulty managing his body, coping with emotions, dealing with relationships, or taking in and processing information. Yet it may not be at all clear *why* the difficulties are present or *how* to address them.

Your child may have difficulties primarily with his *school academic performance*. The school personnel may have several questions:

- Does your child have a problem with learning itself, or an emotional/behavioral disorder which interferes with learning?

- Is there a neurological or medical condition that contributes to the problem?

A psycho-educational evaluation by the school psychologist may be the first step. If that test does not give enough information, school personnel may refer your child for evaluation and testing by an out-of-school child mental health specialist.

Your child may have difficulties primarily with his *school relationships*—with peers and/or adults. The school personnel may have several questions:

- What is contributing to the difficulties?

- What can the adults do to help your child?

- Does your child have a mild learning, attention, or cognitive (thinking) problem that leaves him at increased risk for emotional, social, and behavioral difficulties?

These problems may raise questions that are sometimes too complex to be answered fully by a school psycho-educational evaluation. Thus a referral to an outside specialist for evaluation and testing is an appropriate second step.

Your child may have emotional distress or behavioral difficulties that show up in other areas of life *outside of school*. If so, you may ask your child's doctor or school personnel to arrange an evaluation and testing to help clarify what is going on inside your child.

To further complicate matters, your child may be referred to more than one child care specialist at the same time or even be referred by one specialist to another specialist. Consider these examples:

- Your child's pediatrician may refer your child at the same time to a social worker for a psycho-social evaluation regarding psychotherapy, and to a psychiatrist for an evaluation regarding the use of medication.

- A child psychiatrist, pediatrician, neurologist, or social worker may refer your child to a psychologist for evaluation and testing. This is done to get more information about your child's particular problem and to help choose among different treatment possibilities.

- A psychologist may refer your child to a child psychiatrist or neurologist for evaluation and testing regarding symptoms or psychological test results that might have a neurological cause or require psychiatric medications.

All of these referrals are to get a deeper look into the emotional life, intellectual capacities and/or medical status of your child to figure out what is going on, what treatment is needed, and how best to proceed during treatment.

You will probably not remember most of the detailed information in this chapter, but having read it you will be able to find that information when you need it.

What is involved in evaluation and testing?

Evaluation and testing involve three major steps:

1. a clinical assessment
2. various tests or evaluation materials
3. interpretation of the tests.

All evaluations performed by any child mental health specialist begin with a *clinical assessment*, which involves the following:

*   getting a history of your child's difficulties (usually this is done during an interview with you and talking with your child)
*   reviewing other evaluations and records
*   contacting (with your permission) your child's teacher, pediatrician, etc.

The interview with you and your child about the difficulties may be brief or quite involved, depending on its purpose and how much information the specialist has about your child at the start of the evaluation.

After the clinical assessment, the child mental health expert may use *various tests, or evaluation materials* such as the Conners Attention Deficit Hyperactivity Disorder Scales, used by a psychiatrist, or a WISC IV, used by a psychologist. (I go into more detail on these tests below.) Testing involves using a particular technique or tool to focus on a specific physical or psychological area. Specific tests let specialists look deeper, physically or psychologically, than they are able to do during the clinical assessment. The tests provide tangible data to either confirm or challenge any "hunches" that the specialist had after the interview with you and your child.

After the tests are given, they must be interpreted. *Tests, and the interpretation of tests, are built upon comparison.* The tests have been standardized. This means that when the test was first developed, thousands of people took it. The average response, or result, was considered normal. The non-average response was considered abnormal.

Based on your child's test results, specialists are able to estimate the future path that your child might follow in the specific area being tested. Of course, something might alter that predicted result. For example, imagine that your child tested below average for math proficiency, reading ability, or hand–eye coordination. Your child would likely remain below average in those areas in the future, unless she received remedial training. Similarly, if your child had abnormal results on an EEG (brainwave test: see Table 6.13, p. 181), tests for depression, or tests of hearing, then he would likely continue to have symptoms associated with those abnormal tests unless some unexpected change took place or treatment happened. These general statements are less true for young children with mild difficulties because a young child's impairments do not so easily translate into future problems.

Testing today is becoming more complex. Generally, this means that the specialist can make better recommendations. But it also means more confusion for you and your child. Below, I describe the most common tests and what they test. I hope this gives a framework for understanding what is involved in psychological testing. Whoever does the testing should be able to explain to you in simple language why the test is being done, what is being tested, and what the results mean.

A. Psychological tests

There are five main categories of psychological tests:

1. tests of ability and general intelligence (to evaluate your child's potential)

2. tests of academic performance (to evaluate what your child has actually learned)

3. tests of specific information-processing skills that underlie learning (to evaluate your child's style of learning, strengths, and deficits)

    a. tests of visual–spatial perceptual functioning, including fine motor functions

    b. tests of auditory memory and visual memory

    c. tests of attentional skills

    d. tests of executive function skills (problem-solving abilities)

    e. tests of language skills

4. tests of general emotional development and functioning (to evaluate your child's emotional maturity, plus style of, and skill at, managing emotions)

    a. form questionnaire tests of emotional development

    b. projective tests of emotional development

5. tests for specific categories of emotional and behavioral disorder (to compare your child's symptoms to particular types of problems).

1. TESTS OF ABILITY AND GENERAL INTELLIGENCE

Tests of ability and general intelligence evaluate your child's overall intellectual functioning and estimate your child's potential. Such tests are helpful when your child's current performance is negatively affected by a learning disorder.

Tests identify how your child is at the time the test is given. They tend to be highly reliable in demonstrating that your child has some significant learning problem. But the tests identify how your child is functioning only at that particular time in his development and not what he may grow up to be, especially with good remedial help.

Table 6.1 shows the most common intelligence tests, what your child experiences when taking the test, and what the tests mean.

Until recently, the most common test used in children has been the Wechsler Intelligence Scale for Children (WISC III). The total scores on the two sections of the WISC III are reported as verbal and performance IQ. The two results are most commonly close to one another, e.g. 102 and 99. Wide gaps, typically more than 20 points, may indicate particular kinds of learning disorders and should be discussed

Table 6.1 Tests of ability and general intelligence

Test name	What your child experiences	What the test means
Wechsler Intelligence Scale for Children (WISC IV) first used in 2003 Ages 6–16	*1. Verbal comprehension scale:* Answering questions with the examiner about vocabulary, general knowledge, and the understanding of practical and sociocultural matters. *2. Perceptual reasoning scale:* Making designs with blocks, visual puzzles, and reasoning about pictures. *3. Working memory scale:* Listening and mentally reorganizing numbers and letters, repeating numbers forward and backward, performing mental arithmetic. *4. Processing speed scale:* Matching abstract designs; figuring out and writing down answers to a number–symbol code.	Looks at the four areas that make up a full-scale IQ. Sometimes used as a measure of ability. Useful for comparing one child's abilities and general intelligence with that of other children and with himself (is a child better with verbal/language learning or perceptual/being shown learning?) Testing may point to particular kinds of learning disorders. *1. **Verbal:*** Tests vocabulary, fund of knowledge, comprehension, and reasoning. *2. **Perceptual reasoning:*** Tests non-language-based reasoning and comprehension. *3. **Working memory:*** Tests ability to hold information in mind at one time and work on it. *4. **Processing speed:*** Tests how quickly numbers and symbols can be copied and abstract designs matched. A wide gap between verbal and perceptual reasoning scores may indicate particular kinds of learning disorders.
Wechsler Preschool and Primary Scales of Intelligence (WPPSI)	A WISC-like test for children 4–6½.	Similar to the WISC.
Wechsler Adults Intelligence Scale (WAIS)	A WISC-like test for adolescents 16 years and older.	Similar to the WISC.
Stanford Binet Intelligence Scales (IQ test) Ages 2–23	*1. **Verbal reasoning:*** Answering questions about vocabulary, understanding of practical and sociocultural matters, and recognizing similarities and differences.	The test has a long history of use—more than half a century—to evaluate verbal reasoning, abstract and visual reasoning, quantitative reasoning, and short-term memory. Not all subtests are administered in all ages. Test results provide the ability to compare verbal and non-verbal performance.

Table 6.1 continued

Test name	What your child experiences	What the test means
	2. Abstract/visual reasoning: Making designs using blocks; copying designs, using logic to find missing piece in pictures or designs, and identifying shapes in folded paper.	
	3. Quantitative reasoning: Using paper and pencil to do math tests; classifying numbers, and doing other number and math activities.	
	4. Short-term memory: Replicating sequences of beads of four shapes and three colors; repeating sentences and digits, and pointing to picture sequences.	
Woodcock–Johnson Cognitive Battery Ages 2–90	Doing such things as: answering questions about pictures, listening to an audiotape and then responding to questions about what was heard, and using paper and pencil for tasks like circling numbers that are the same or tracing a pattern.	This is a newer test being used in various parts of the USA. There are 21 different subtests and measures of seven abilities, including visual and auditory speed of processing, long-term and short-term memory, comprehension, fund of knowledge, and fluid reasoning.

and explained by your child's examiner during the meeting in which you are told about the results of the testing.

The WISC IV is rapidly replacing the WISC III. It is thought to provide better assessment of a child's raw ability to learn (fluid reasoning), working memory, and processing speed, as well as being more culturally fair. Some psychologists worry that the three subtests of the perceptual reasoning scale on WISC IV might not always give as accurate a picture as the WISC III performance scale of some children with non-verbal learning disorder (NVLD) or Asperger's disorder. If questions arise about the accuracy of WISC IV test results, get a second opinion.

This new version (WISC IV) has four scales that make up a full-scale IQ, rather than only two scales (primary subtests are in parentheses):

1. verbal comprehension (similarities, vocabulary, and comprehension)
2. perceptual reasoning (matrix reasoning, block design, picture concepts)
3. working memory (letter-numbers sequencing, digit span)
4. processing speed (symbol search, coding).

For each scale additional tests may be substituted for the primary subtests.

An experienced psychologist can use the WISC, WPPSI, or WAIS to estimate your child's specific learning skills difficulties and some underlying capacities. These estimates may be confirmed or disproved by the tests listed in Section 3, below.

2. TESTS OF ACADEMIC PERFORMANCE

Tests of academic performance evaluate how your child is doing relative to where she would be expected to be, given her age and grade. These tests do not measure ability; they measure academic skills and knowledge that your child has learned.

Understanding academic and other tests scores

Most tests scores are shown either as *percentiles* or as *standard scores*. You can understand *percentiles* by thinking of placing your child's score within a group of 100. For example, if your child has a score at the 60th percentile, it means that of 100 children taking the test, 59 of them would score lower than your child and 40 would score higher. For most tests, an average score will be between the 25th and the 75th percentile.

A *standard* score on a test is structured, or "calibrated," so that the midpoint score of the test is set at either 50 or 100. Scores higher or lower than that midpoint may be expressed as "standard deviations." This is a measure of the distance a score is from the average score. Standard deviations divide the score into broad categories. For example, if your child scores 100, she might be exactly in the midpoint (where the average score has been set). If she scores 115, she might be one standard deviation higher than average. With an 85, she might be one standard deviation lower than the average score. A result of two standard deviations below the average would indicate your child is significantly behind.

Usually, educational tests have an *age equivalent* or *grade equivalent score*. This indicates the age or grade level at which most children got that same score. Suppose your child is in the eighth month of third grade, or "3:8." On a reading test, she gets a "grade" score of 2:7. This means that she is reading at the level that is average for a child in the seventh month of the second grade—about a year below her actual grade. Test results of two years below your child's expected level are considered an indication of a learning disorder. More specific testing (see Section 3 below) will help sort out which of the possible causes are contributing to your child being below grade level.

Some psychological and educational tests can be machine-scored, using software that produces a report. Although such results come quickly and fairly inexpensively, they are no substitute for a comprehensive report written by a specialist who administers the tests.

- A psychologist integrates parents' and teachers' observations with her own observations of how your child performs during the test.

- The psychologist evaluates how the results are connected to one another, and then draws important conclusions about your child's functioning.

- The psychologist relates all the findings to the specific concerns of parents' and teachers' that led to the evaluation.

The psychologist compares how your child responds to the tests with the many other children she has observed doing the same activity. Very crucial understanding can often only come from such observations.

Table 6.2 outlines some of the common tests of academic performance.

Table 6.2 Tests of academic performance

Test name	What your child experiences	What the test means
The Woodcock–Johnson Tests of Achievement Ages 2–90	Reading and writing. Reading single words, made up words that test phonics, and sentences in order to supply a missing word. Writing spelling tests and mathematics tests for doing calculations and problem solving (both timed and untimed).	Reviews broad academic areas and compares an individual child to others of the same age and grade. Results are given as age and grade equivalent scores and percentile ranking.
Wide Range Achievement Test (WRAT) Ages 5–75	Reading single words and doing paper and pencil tests of spelling and numerical calculations. Takes 20–30 minutes to complete.	Tests reading recognition, spelling, and arithmetic. Results can be compared with IQ and grade equivalents as a screening measurement of achievement.
Wechsler Individual Achievement Test (WIAT) Ages 4–85	Reading single words, made up words to test phonic capacities; a passage, and then answering questions about it for up to 15 minutes. Then listening to a story and answering questions about it. Responding to questions about math concepts; performing calculations.	Gives information about academic skills and problem-solving ability. Tests basic skills for reading, spelling, writing, listening, comprehension and oral expression, and math. It may be linked to WISC IV.
Woodcock Diagnostic Reading Battery Ages 2+	Reading single words, made up words to test for phonic capacities, and sentences which must have a missing word supplied. Reading as many simple sentences as possible within a time limit.	Breaks reading into some of its components: reading comprehension, and word comprehension, recognition, and analysis. Provides a comparative look at skills within a child and in comparison to others.

Continued on next page

Table 6.2 continued

Test name	What your child experiences	What the test means
Nelson–Denny Reading Test Grades 9 through college	Taking a multiple-choice vocabulary test and a comprehension test that involves reading passages and answering multiple-choice questions about them. Both sections have time limits.	Used to assess a student's qualifications and need for extended time on academic tasks, as it provides measures for standard and extended test-taking times. The College Board requires this test for disability determination.
Gray Oral Reading Test Ages 6–18.11 months	Reading paragraphs of increasing difficulty out loud and then answering multiple-choice questions read to child. Takes 20–30 minutes.	Assesses reading fluency, rate, accuracy, and comprehension. It helps identify oral reading difficulties and measures improvement.
Key Math Test Ages 5–22	Doing math problems in head and using paper and pencil.	Measures skill of math concepts and operations including: applications with whole numbers and fractions; geometry, measurement; time and money; estimation; interpreting data and problem-solving.

Some examiners prefer using the WIAT test of achievement along with the WISC test of ability. They believe that this combination allows for more valid information because the tests have been standardized together. Remember, these tests of achievement assess what has been learned: academic skills and knowledge. **Wide discrepancies between the earlier ability tests and these academic tests call for further investigation**.

3. TESTS OF SPECIFIC INFORMATION-PROCESSING SKILLS WHICH UNDERLIE LEARNING

When an imbalance is found between your child's potential abilities (Table 6.1, p. 164) and how he is performing (Table 6.2, above), additional tests to assess your child's information processing may be needed. These tests evaluate specific capacities:

- hand–eye coordination with paper and pencil
- auditory or visual learning and memory (how your child takes in and remembers what he hears and sees)
- attention (being aware and concentrating)
- executive functions (abilities needed to plan, organize, and complete a task)
- visual–auditory perception (the ability to decode the written word)
- phonological processing (the ability to hear phonics/word sounds).

These and other capacities or skills, like those identified with the Wechsler tests, are cognitive functions: abilities that make up thinking and learning. The results of these tests can identify your child's specific disability with thinking and learning.

The underlying cause of the disability might be in one or more cognitive skills. For example, your child may have reading problems or difficulty with learning mathematics. The underlying cause may be a problem in the cognitive skill of short-term auditory or visual memory, in understanding what is being said, or in making use of what is understood. These disabilities are usually independent of the teaching or materials used in school with your child. But if your child's disabilities are not addressed by school resources, the situation can get worse over time. If, by contrast, your child receives proper remediation, he can learn to compensate for his disability and to function more effectively.

Tests of specific informational processing skills are usually not part of a routine psycho-educational school battery (a group of tests used together). When these tests (like those listed in Tables 6.5–6.8) *are* included, along with general tests of ability (Table 6.1, above) and performance (Table 6.2, above), it is called a *neuropsychological evaluation*. This provides detailed knowledge of your child's learning and thinking (cognitive) patterns and allows a closer evaluation of the specific information-processing abilities underlying learning.

A neuropsychologist chooses and administers these tests of specific information processing. Neuropsychologists are doctoral level psychologists (PhD, PsyD, or EdD) with special training in these more complex tests for assessing cognitive function. The neuropsychologist chooses which tests to use based on the understanding of your child's patterns which came from the results of the tests of abilities and intelligence (above).

In some parts of the USA, the two tests in Table 6.3 are commonly all that may be used for neuropsychological testing.

In contrast to using the preceding "battery approach" to testing, many neuropsychologists, particularly in the Northeast, use a "process approach" to testing. This means that the examiner chooses, from a wide array of tests, the particular tests that best fit each individual child. The subtests from the Wechsler Intelligence Scale for Children (WISC IV, in Category 1, above) give important preliminary information in the five specific areas that follow: visual–spatial, auditory and visual memory, attention, executive function, language. With this and other information, the psychologist chooses particular areas and tests for a child to use. Remember that any one test may evaluate many different types of basic functioning. All of the tests below help to clarify reading, writing, or math problems and also provide information about behavioral and social difficulties.

Different examiners may use different tests. No single test can answer all questions. And no child would be tested in all the areas listed below: it would be

Table 6.3 Commonly used groups of tests for neuropsychological evaluation

Test name	What your child experiences	What the test means
Halstead–Reitan Battery Ages 8–adult	Engages in many different types of activities such as: listening to musical patterns and differentiating between them; drawing lines to connect dots in a certain order; using index finger to tap a bar as quickly as the child is able; placing textured pegs into holes on a pegboard.	Gives one combined score that measures brain dysfunction. Consists of a set of 10 comprehensive neuropsychological tests that examines language, attention, motor speed, abstract thinking, memory, and spatial reasoning. Some neuropsychologists use a few or all of the original set of tests in this battery.
Luria–Nebraska Neuropsychological Battery, Children's Revision Ages 15+	Engages in many different types of activities such as: telling a story in response to a picture; copying a shape embedded in a larger shape; telling how two things are similar or different; remembering a rhythmic sequence; responding to the examiner's verbal or motor cues with particular alternate cues. Takes 1.5–2.5 hours.	Comparable to Halstead–Reitan, this is a set of 14 tests that covers a broad range of spheres of performance (including assessment of right and left brain functions) and provides analyses of strengths and weakness across different areas of brain function.

Table 6.4 Tests of visual–spatial perceptual functioning

Test name	What your child experiences	What the test means
Bender Visual Motor Gestalt Test Ages 4+	Copying nine geometric designs that your child is shown, one at a time. Takes ten minutes.	Used to assess the ability to organize and copy visual stimuli into whole patterns. The number and type of errors your child makes are scored and compared with standards developed for children of a similar age.
Beery Test of Visual Motor Integration Short Format for ages 2–15	Copying drawings of geometric forms arranged in order of increasing difficulty.	Helps assess the extent to which individuals can integrate their visual and motor abilities. Your child's copies of the forms are compared with standards developed for children of a similar age.
Rey–Osterrieth Complex Figure Test Ages 5+	Copying a complicated figure and later drawing it from memory.	Helps to identify how well and in what way your child organizes what he sees.

burdensome on your child and take too much time. Below I describe some of the more common tests for neuropsychological evaluation used throughout the USA.

a. Tests of visual–spatial perceptual functioning, including fine motor functions

This set of tests usually involves drawing. The tests help the examiner to see whether or not, as well as how, your child can copy what he sees.

b. Tests of auditory memory and visual memory functioning

These tests help clarify reading problems or other learning difficulties your child has.

Table 6.5 Tests of auditory memory and visual memory functioning

Test name	What your child experiences	What the test means
Wide Range Assessment of Memory and Learning (WRAML) Ages 5–90	Retelling a story told by the examiner and repeating sentences. Copying designs from memory, replicating spatial sequences of increasing length, and learning visual and verbal information. Takes about 45 minutes.	Measures working memory and short-term memory for visual and verbal information, attention and concentration, recall and recognition after 20 minutes. There are six core tests: (1) verbal memory (story memory and verbal learning), (2) visual memory (design memory), (3) attention/concentration memory, (4) working memory, (5) verbal recognition memory, (6) visual recognition memory.
Wechsler Children's Memory Scale Ages 5–16	Being given various kinds of information: a paragraph of reading material, paired words, pictures of scenes, pictures of faces, various word sequences, etc. and then being asked to recall the information—sometimes with details, sometimes not—immediately and after a short delay. Takes 30–35 minutes of testing and 25–30 minutes between sections to complete all the material.	Looks at attention and working memory, verbal and visual memory, short- and long-delay memory, recall and recognition, and specific learning characteristics. The examiner can use the results to compare a child's memory and learning to his ability, attention, and achievement as shown on the Wechsler Intelligence Scale for Children and Wechsler Individual Achievement Test.
California Verbal Learning Test—Children's Version Ages 5–16 years 11 months	Being read a list and then saying as many words that can be remembered, both immediately and after a 20-minute delay.	Examines several aspects of verbal learning, learning strategies/organization, and memory/recall.
Rey–Osterrieth Complex Figure Test	See Table 6.4	See Table 6.4

Other tests mentioned earlier also give information about memory. For example, the academic tests (Table 6.2, above) may indicate whether your child has memorized knowledge, can remember the sequences of procedures (like when doing long division), and can retrieve that knowledge on demand.

c. Tests of attentional skills

These tests help clarify difficulties in noticing, concentrating, and paying attention that may interfere with learning and contribute to behavioral problems in and out of school. The term *executive function difficulties* is commonly used to describe problems with attention, organization, and planning associated with learning disorders and attentional disorders (attention deficit hyperactivity disorder (ADHD)).

Computer tests like the Conners' CPT and the TOVA (Table 6.6, below) give some objective measure of your child's problem with attention, as well as with distractibility and impulsivity. These tests are used more often to monitor the response to medication treatment of an attentional skill deficit rather than simply to identify it.

To assess whether your child has attention ADHD, the preceding tests are used, plus various checklists and questionnaires, such as the Conners' Scales (see Table 6.11, below). Such testing does help to diagnose ADHD. But the most important factor in accurately diagnosing ADHD is to have a detailed review of your child's earlier development and the current observations, recorded on questionnaires and inventories, which you and your child's teachers make.

Questionnaires (lists of questions to be responded to) and inventories (lists of symptoms to be check marked) that focus on the central symptoms of inattention and distractibility, hyperactivity, and impulsivity can be used periodically to measure progress. Psychological and neuropsychological tests help identify learning disabilities and emotional problems that can occur along with ADHD.

d. Tests of executive function skills (problem-solving abilities)

These tests look at difficulties in initiating, planning, and organizing information. They also test working memory (the ability to hold information in mind while performing complex tasks), flexibility, goal-directed persistence, and time management. The tests of executive function can indicate why your child has learning difficulties.

e. Tests of language skills

These can help clarify specific problems in language development and usage. Children with problems in language might have problems in classroom participation and learning. Many excellent tests are used to assess language. In Table 6.8 (below) I describe some common ones.

Table 6.6 Tests of attention

Test name	What your child experiences	What the test means
Subtests of the WISC (ability test) and subtests of the WRAML (achievement test)	See Tables 6.1 and 6.4	Used to assess attentional skills.
Trail Making Test, part A and B Ages 6+	Connecting dots on a piece of paper by number and letter, using a pencil.	Measures attention, visual planning, visual sequencing, planning, inhibition, set shifting, and mental flexibility. This test is sensitive to global brain status but is not too sensitive to minor brain injuries.
Conners' CPT (continuous performance test) Ages 4+	Sitting at a computer and performing a task that involves pressing a mouse button, or keyboard spacebar, when certain letters appear on the monitor and not pressing when different letters appear. Letters are presented at varying intervals.	It requires intense attention to a visual–motor task, assesses sustained attention and freedom from distractibility.
Test of Variable Attention (TOVA) Ages 6+. Shorter version: Ages 4–5	Sitting at a computer and performing a task that consists of repeated exposures to two different types of squares. Pressing a button every time a particular type of square is flashed on the monitor screen. Takes about 22 minutes; a shorter version takes 11 minutes.	Measures errors of omission (inattention) and commission (impulsivity) and is used in the diagnosis and monitoring of the treatment of ADHD. An ADHD score, which is a comparison to an age/gender-specific ADHD group, is provided.
NEPSY Ages 3–12	Doing hands-on tasks, such as using blocks and balls to solve problems. (This format is particularly appealing to young children.) Listening to an audiotape and responding to questions by pointing to a picture that represents a specific word or picking up a color square that is asked for. Drawing geometric forms or crossing out target images using paper and pencil.	Evaluates five areas: attention/executive functions, sensorimotor functioning, visuospatial processing, memory, and learning. It can be helpful in identifying children with learning disabilities, ADHD, autistic-type disorders, and speech and language impairments.

Table 6.7 Tests of executive function

Test name	What your child experiences	What the test means
Bender-Gestalt and subtests of the WISC	See Tables 6.1 (WISC) and 6.4 (Bender)	Provides a general assessment of your child's executive function abilities.
Trail Making Test, part A and B	Connecting dots on a piece of paper by number and letter, using a pencil.	Measures attention, visual planning, visual sequencing, planning, inhibition, set shifting, and mental flexibility. This test is sensitive to overall brain condition but is not too sensitive to minor brain injuries.
Delis–Kaplan Executive Functions System (D–KEFS) Ages 8–89	Engaging in an interesting game-like format that does not provide right or wrong feedback.	Assesses key areas of executive function (problem-solving, thinking flexibility, fluency of thinking, planning, inhibition, and deductive reasoning) in both spatial and verbal abstract thinking. Believed to be a measure of frontal lobe function.
Wisconsin Card Sort Test Ages 6.5+	Being asked to figure out rules concerning the arrangement of cards of different shapes and colors.	Measures non-verbal problem-solving and other cognitive abilities. This procedure also measures the ability to learn concepts and mental flexibility. Considered a good measure of frontal lobe functioning.
Booklet Category Test Ages 5+	Looking at letters, shapes, and designs then identifying what's common in a group.	Measures non-verbal problem-solving and reasoning, rule learning, hypothesis testing, concept learning, and mental flexibility.
NEPSY Ages 3–12	See Table 6.6	See Table 6.6
Tower of London Test Ages 7+	Moving and placing wooden discs from one vertical dowel to another to complete the Tower of London.	Assesses higher-level problem-solving, rule learning, spatial planning, impulsivity, and concentration.
Stroop Test Ages 5+	Looking at a series of cards and (following directions) reading words and naming colors.	Measures focus, attention, concentration, set shifting, and inhibition (capacities of executive function), as well as mental flexibility and vitality.

Table 6.8 Tests of language

Test name	What your child experiences	What the test means
Clinical Evaluation of Language Fundamentals Ages 5–21	Responding to spoken questions by pointing to pictures and words, or responding with sentences to pictures and spoken words.	Tests ability to understand (receptive language) and express ideas (expressive language) through a series of interactive tasks.
Comprehensive Assessment of Spoken Language Ages 3–21	Answering questions in a variety of verbal activities.	Tests for the identification, diagnosis, and follow-up evaluation of language and expressive and receptive communication disorders.
Boston Naming Test Ages 6+	Being shown 60 line-drawn pictures of common objects (comb, house, etc.) and saying what each is.	Uncovers problems with naming things/word retrieval and is useful when evaluating children with learning disabilities.
Peabody Picture Vocabulary Test Ages: 2.6–90+	Being shown a page with a number of black and white pictures of different objects and actions and pointing to the object or action being named. For example, "Which one is mowing?"	Tests receptive vocabulary achievement and verbal ability in English-speaking individuals. It is used to assess receptive (hearing) vocabulary and as a screening test for verbal ability.
Comprehensive Test of Phonological Processing (CTOPP) Ages: 5.0—24.11	Listening to sounds and being asked questions about the child's awareness of a sound, about ability to remember having heard a sound, and to identify a sound.	Assesses the ability to separate and combine sounds, an essential component of early reading. Persons with deficits in one or more of these kinds of phonological processing abilities may have more difficulty learning to read than those who do not.

4. TESTS OF GENERAL EMOTIONAL DEVELOPMENT AND FUNCTIONING

The preceding tests focus primarily on identifying learning, attention, and various cognitive disorders. But your child may have emotional, social, and adjustment problems because of those cognitive disabilities. Thus, when a psychologist is evaluating a child who has a primary learning disorder, he or she might include tests of general emotional development and functioning just as he or she uses them to assess a child whose problem is primarily emotional or behavioral.

These tests may be divided into two groups:

a. *Form questionnaire tests* have questions that require unambiguous answers, such as "yes," "no," "never," "frequently," etc.

- Usually the form is filled out by your child, you, or the examiner.

- The form is then scored (often by computer).

- Only a little experience is needed to give this first group of tests.

b. *Projective tests* can have a wide range of answers. For example, a child might be shown an unformed image and say, "It looks like a bat," or be shown a distinct image and say, "The boy (in the picture) is sad because he disappointed his father."

- The test is given and interpreted by someone with expertise. I discuss both types of tests below.

a. Form questionnaire tests of emotional development

The first two form questionnaires in Table 6.9 have a long history and are used quite frequently. The Behavior Assessment System for Children, a newer test, is being used with increasing frequency.

The test results for the Minnesota Multiphasic Personality Inventory for adolescents and the Millon Adolescent Clinical Inventory are often interpreted by computer. Much training and clinical experience are required to make more than superficial meaning of the computer-generated report. A Millon score report presented without such clinical judgment in its interpretation may be quite misleading.

b. Projective tests of emotional development

Projective tests are based upon the idea that a person who is shown a picture or design that has no particular meaning to it will assign a meaning to it that reflects that person's own personal experience. For example, in the Hand Test (not described in Table 6.10), an examiner presents pictures of hands in various positions. Then the viewer is asked to say what the hands are doing or to make up a story about what the hands are doing.

5. TESTS FOR SPECIFIC CATEGORIES OF EMOTIONAL AND BEHAVIORAL DISORDERS

These tests use questions that focus on a particular set of symptoms, that is, particular disorders. The questionnaire tests listed below may be administered or scored by individuals without any special training. Those that involve interviewing and observation require training. Examples of the different types of tests are provided in Table 6.11.

Table 6.9 Form questionnaires to test emotional development

Test name	What your child experiences	What the test means
Minnesota Multiphasic Personality Inventory (MMPI) Ages 13+	Filling out a questionnaire that involves a long series of questions with true/false type answers.	Helps address problems clinicians are more likely to see with adolescents, such as family issues, eating disorders, and chemical dependency. This assessment of personality and emotional status is often used along with various neuropsychological tests and can increase understanding about the reactions to brain impairment.
Millon Adolescent Clinical Inventory Ages 13–18	Filling out a questionnaire with true/false type answers.	Evaluates a number of personality characteristics. Your adolescent's responses are compared with the responses of others who have identifiable patterns of particular personality characteristics and emotional disturbance. A specialist needs a great deal of training and clinical experience to interpret these tests accurately and make deeper meaning of the computer-generated report.
Children's Personality Questionnaire Ages 8–12	Parent responds to a list of brief descriptions of behavior. For example, the list may include "bites nails." The choices for response are "never," "sometimes," "often," and "everyday."	Measures 14 primary personality traits that are useful in understanding and evaluating a pre-adolescent's personal, social, and academic development. Results include narrative interpretations on topics such as creativity, emotional stability, self-concept level, excitability, apprehension, and extraversion.
Parents' rating scales of the Behavior Assessment System for Children (BASC) Ages 4–18	Parents and/or teachers complete a questionnaire about a child's behavior and symptoms at home and in school. It takes 10 to 20 minutes.	Consists of five measures intended to gather information from a variety of sources (teacher, parent, direct student observation, student self-report, and structured developmental history), which may be used individually or in any combination. Designed to assess and identify children and adolescents with emotional disturbances and behavioral disorders.

Table 6.10 Projective tests of emotional development

Test name	What your child experiences	What the test means
Rorschach (named after the test creator, Hermann Rorschach)	Looking at ten standardized cards, each with a different ink blot design, and then reporting any shapes, forms, or images that the child identifies in these designs.	Based upon the pattern of your child's responses, a skilled interpreter/psychologist can infer signs of emotional disturbance, and strength, as well as personality structure.
Adolescent Apperception Ages 12–19	Being shown 11 cards with pictures that focus on parent, peer, and sibling interaction and then creating a story from each card.	Provides a non-intrusive way to obtain information concerning feelings about self and others.
Children's Apperception Test Ages 3–10	Being shown ten card scenes showing a variety of animal figures, mostly in unmistakably human social settings, and then creating a story from each card.	Based on the assumption that young children would find it easier to talk about appealing drawings of animals than drawings of humans.
Kinetic Drawing System for Family and School Ages 3+	Being asked to draw something specific: a picture of the child's family, or of a person doing something.	The evaluator asks your child about the drawing and uses some standardized guides to provide general conclusions, and occasionally specific ones, regarding the child's emotional life.
House–Tree–Person Drawing Test Ages 3+	Being asked to draw a house, a tree, and a person.	
Human Figure Drawing Ages 3+	Being asked to draw a person.	

B. Non-psychological tests

The following tests may be sought because findings on psychological evaluation need more specialized assessment. Or the idea of such assessments may come up after a clinical evaluation by your child's doctor, therapist, or school staff.

1. TESTS FOR EVIDENCE OF SPECIFIC SENSORY OR MOTOR DISORDERS

A psychologist who administers any of the tests described may note a deficit in your child's *speech and language*. However, usually a *speech pathologist* (an expert in the area of speech and language) provides a definitive diagnosis and treatment plan. Your child may also undergo a range of specific tests, including evaluation of his hearing.

Table 6.11 Tests for specific categories of emotional and behavioral functioning

Test name	What your child experiences	What the test means
Children's Depression Rating Scale (CDRS-R) Ages 6-12	Asked questions by an interviewer that covers 17 items. Takes 15-20 minutes.	Evaluates severity of a depressed mood, covering five symptom areas of depression.
Children's Depression Inventory (CDI) Ages 6-17	Answers questions in a paper and pencil format about feelings over the preceding two weeks. Chooses the best of three choices offered for each of 27 questions. Takes 10 minutes. Administered individually or in groups.	Evaluates the severity of a depressed mood covering five symptom areas.
Revised Children's Manifest Anxiety Scale(RCMAS) Ages 6+	Asked questions, with yes or no response, by an interviewer that covers 28 Items. Takes 5 minutes	Evaluates severity of anxiety.
YBOCS (Yale–Brown obsessive–compulsive scale) Ages 6+	Being asked ten questions about various behaviors and inner experiences. The test has been converted recently to self-report format and scored on a computer.	Assesses the severity of obsessions and compulsions, independent of the number and type of obsessions or compulsions present.
Conners' Attention Deficit Hyperactivity Disorder Scales Ages 3–17	Teacher, parent, and child fill out separate questionnaire forms, which contain ADHD-related and non-ADHD-related symptoms rated on a 0–3 scale. It takes 20 minutes or less.	Assesses for ADHD and conduct problems, cognitive problems, family problems, and emotional problems such as anger control and anxiety.
Autism Diagnostic Observation Scale (ADOS) All ages and levels	Engaging in specific kinds of activities while being observed for the occurrence, or non-occurrence, of behaviors that have been identified as important to the diagnosis of autism and other pervasive developmental disorders.	Evaluates communication, social interaction, play, and the imaginative use of materials.
Childhood Autism Rating Scales (CARS) Ages 2–adult	*Parents* are interviewed, or an evaluator observes your child, for levels of general developmental skills, socialization skills, and coping skills.	Identifies children with autism and distinguishes them from developmentally handicapped children who are not autistic.
Asperger's syndrome diagnostic test (ASDS) Ages 5–18	Anyone who knows your child or adolescent (*parents, teachers, siblings, psychiatrists, and other professionals*) completes this yes–no 50 item scale. Takes 10–15 minutes.	Identifies the presence of Asperger's syndrome through the assessment of cognitive functioning, maladaptive behaviors, language, sensory motor and social functioning.

Many checklists/scales do not focus on one specific category of disorder, but assess for a whole range of disorders (Table 6.12).

Table 6.12 Tests for a range of childhood emotional and behavioral disorders

Test name	What your child experiences	What the test means
Achenbach Child Behavior Checklist Ages 4–18	Parents fill out a form with 118 questions about their child's behavioral problems and social abilities which are scored on a three-point scale: "not true, true, often true."	Focuses on a select range of specific disorders. There are five scale scores. It is designed to assess, in a standardized way, the behavioral problems and social competencies of children as reported by parents.
Children's Interview for Psychiatric Syndromes (ChIPS) Ages 6–18	Parents and older children (adolescents) are interviewed for about 30 minutes in a highly structured format with simple language questions related to symptoms of 20 psychiatric disorders.	Screens for 20 disorders, as well as psychological and social stressors.
Personality Inventory for Children (PIC) Ages 5–19	Parents, child and teacher each fill out a 275 true–false item questionnaire. It takes about 40 minutes.	Assesses for cognitive impairment, family dysfunction, psychological discomfort, impulsivity and distractibility, reality distortion, social withdrawal, delinquency, somatic concern, social skill deficits. Together the scales provide an integrated picture of a child's adjustment at home, at school, and in the community.
Behavior Assessment System for Children (BASC)	See Table 6.9	See Table 6.9

Your child may have a hard time managing his body. This may be due to a deficit in *motor and/or sensory functioning*. Particularly in younger children, problems caused by impaired motor (muscle) or sensory integration may go along with or contribute to emotional and behavioral difficulties.

Your child may have problems with *fine motor functioning* (the actions of the fingers, hand, and arm), for example, the ability to draw, write, and play a musical instrument. If so, an *occupational therapist* OT may provide diagnosis and treatment. Occupational therapists also assess and treat a problem identified as sensory integration dysfunction. The OT assessment, perhaps using the Sensory Integration and Praxis Tests (SIPT), includes an evaluation of your child's senses of sight, sound, smell, taste, and the various modalities of touch: pain, temperature, pressure, and movement. The evaluation looks closely at how your child's sensitivities in the different sensory areas impact on such activities as motor, social, educational, and emotional functioning. An occupational therapist is skilled in the use of various activities that help with your child's physical and emotional rehabilitation.

To evaluate and treat problems primarily in motor functioning, a *physical therapist* (a specialist in motor strength and motor coordination disorders) may work with your child. A physical therapist is an expert in problems that involve large muscle groups that enable a child to run, dance, and hit a ball.

2. TESTS FOR EVIDENCE OF A MEDICAL DISORDER

Generally, lab or instrument tests are not performed unless there is some indication of a possible medical disorder (based on information gathered during the clinical evaluation by the pediatrician, neurologist, psychiatrist, or testing by the psychologist).

Table 6.13 Tests for medical causes of psychological disorders

Test name	What your child experiences	What the test means
Blood tests	Blood is drawn and microscopically looked at for abnormalities that indicate medical disorders.	Checks for problems such as thyroid disease, diabetes, or anemia that could cause emotional and behavioral difficulties.
EEG	A brainwave test that assesses, painlessly, whether the electrical activity of the brain is normal or not.	Used if there is reason to believe that your child's emotional, behavioral, or learning problems result from an irregularity of brain electrical function.
MRI, CAT scan, SPECT	Creates computer-aided images of the brain.	Only used if there is a specific sign that your child's problem might result from a brain abnormality (such as an injury to the brain tissue, a tumor, or deformity) that could be seen on these tests.

Who *does* the testing and who *wants* the information?
Who does *the testing?*

The first tests to assess for a learning disorder are usually administered by a *psychologist* with at least a master's level in school psychology or in clinical psychology. This first evaluation would include tests for general intelligence testing/ability (WISC IV, etc. in A1, above), for general academic performance/achievement (WRAT, etc. in A2 above), and for specific academic (math/reading) skills (Nelson–Denny, Key Math in A2, above).

The more complex tests to assess cognitive function, which look at specific information-processing abilities underlying learning (Bender, Rey–Osterrieth, Delis–Kaplan etc. in A3 above), are usually performed by doctoral level *psychologists* (PhD, PsyD, or EdD), who have had additional training in neuropsychology and are referred to as *neuropsychologists*. Insurance companies do not often pay for this more complex testing unless there is a specific medical or psychiatric/mental disorder that is being investigated.

The screening tests of general emotional development and functioning (MMPI, projective tests, etc. in A4 above) are performed by *school counselors* or *psychologists* who have at least a master's degree, but more often a doctorate. The more complicated projective tests of emotional development usually require the skill and training of a doctoral level psychologist. The tests for specific categories of emotional and behavioral functioning (depression, anxiety, and ADHD scales, etc. in A5 above) may be used by any specialist—*psychiatrist, psychologist, neurologist, or pediatrician*—during the initial evaluation.

Speech and language pathologists, occupational therapists, and physical therapists perform tests related to their specific areas. Medical tests and the EEG test may be ordered by any physician. The EEG test results are usually interpreted only by a *neurologist*.

Who wants *the information?*

If your child has a learning difficulty, then *you*, the *classroom teacher, special education personnel*, and other school staff all want to know more about the causes of your child's problems. They would want your child tested for a specific learning disorder and for the presence of ADHD. Such symptoms, like inattention and distractibility, as well as hyperactivity and impulsivity, may be contributing significantly to your child's learning difficulty. With good information, your child's teachers then can choose methods of instruction that are specific to your child's problem. And the *school counseling staff* will be better able to work with your child to address emotional and behavioral problems.

Similarly, a *mental health professional* treating your child would find various psychological tests useful:

- Results of psychological testing that assesses general emotional development (MMPI or Mellon) can illuminate your child's emotional strengths and vulnerabilities.

- Cognitive tests revealing information about language processing and capacity for abstract thinking help with planning and focusing treatment.

- Projective psychological testing, along with questionnaires for specific categories of emotional difficulties, provide understanding about the nature and extent of your child's emotional problems and strengths that can help guide pharmacotherapy as well as psychotherapy.

Since complex psychological tests are so expensive, they generally are used only for more complicated and confusing emotional and behavioral problems. When more complex testing is not available, the tests for specific categories of emotional and behavioral functioning that have accompanying interpretations of results built into the test (depression, anxiety, and ADHD, etc. scales in A5 above) may be administered by a psychologist, psychiatrist, or social worker and used to guide treatment.

A physician may want medical or neurological tests as he investigates and treats emotional, behavioral, or learning problems in your child.

Table 6.14 Who does the evaluations?

Specialist	Administers and interprets complex tests for learning, emotional, and behavioral difficulties. Tests A1–4	Administers scales and simple tests for specific categories of emotional and behavioral difficulties. Tests A5	Orders and interprets medical tests for learning, emotional, and behavioral difficulties. Tests B2
Psychologist	Yes	Yes	No
Psychiatrist	No	Yes	Yes
Neurologist	No	Yes	Yes
Pediatrician	No	Yes	Yes

Where is the evaluation done?

Usually the testing is done at the office of the person giving the tests. Two practical distinctions are important. The first distinction is between testing that is done *within the school system* and testing done *outside the school system*. Most school systems have psychologists who can administer general intelligence tests, academic performance tests, tests of specific academic skills, and some simple projective tests. An educational specialist, usually the special education teacher, also assesses academic performance and skills. This in-school testing is part of the psycho-educational assessment.

Sometimes more complex testing is needed to clarify a problem and determine treatment needs. A child then may be referred to someone in the community with the skills and experience to perform those more complex tests. Often school systems pay for this testing. However, financial responsibility varies by state. Refer to the special education laws and regulations for your state. Given that school budgets are quite tight these days, school personnel may resist referring your child for outside testing. As a parent you may need to advocate strongly for further testing, especially if the plan based upon the in-school testing doesn't seem to be working for your child.

The second distinction is between testing done by *several different private specialists* and testing done by a *team of specialists affiliated with a hospital or medical center*. Individual specialists may be quite competent. But I believe that people working together and doing evaluations on a daily basis are likely to have better communication than those who do not. Complex situations often require several different kinds of specialists: neurologist, child psychiatrist, psychologist, pediatrician, speech pathologist, and occupational therapist. When a parent wants a clear picture of a child with a very complicated problem, the communication between the multiple specialists is crucial. Thus, in such cases, I recommend a team approach.

A clinical example

Below is an example of the "why, what, and who" of a neuropsychological evaluation.

David was an unhappy eight and a half-year-old boy referred for a psychological evaluation by the school staff and his parents. He was increasingly discontented in school and had begun to avoid school work. His teacher said that David had problems focusing and attending, especially with difficult work. His mind seemed to wander a lot and he missed much of what his teacher said. The more difficult the work, the more he seemed to be in his own world.

David had trouble with writing. His handwriting was so sloppy that sometimes even he couldn't read it. One day he burst into tears when the kids teased him because he couldn't read the words he had written on the board. David could communicate verbally but often did not notice inaccuracies in his use of spoken and written language. He had difficulty responding to his teacher's directions appropriately. He also had difficulty organizing and estimating the time and proper sequence needed to complete a given task. He appeared immature and somewhat manipulative.

At home, David's parents saw that he did not want to read and preferred to watch television. He had trouble following a story. He also had difficulty with friendships: he was isolated both in and outside of school. His tendency to "space out" made him seem less present and interested in what was happening around him. Other students shied away from asking him to get involved in an activity. He was sensitive to rejection.

David's parents met with the school staff, hoping to have a psycho-educational evaluation in school. But the school psychologist was ill and would not return for several months. Given that David's troubles were getting worse, his parents did not want to wait and requested that their son start directly with an outside psychologist. The school administration agreed and arranged the evaluation.

David's parents met with a local clinical psychologist who specialized in neuropsychological evaluations. The psychologist spent time with David's parents to gather historical information about David that would help her evaluate his current level of cognitive and behavioral functioning. She then talked with David for about half an hour before beginning the tests which lasted about six hours over the course of three days. At that meeting, and two other meetings, she conducted her formal evaluation.

- To evaluate his general ability and intelligence (his potential), she used the Wechsler Intelligence Scale for Children. He scored a total IQ of 110, in the high average range.
- To evaluate his achievements (what he's actually learned), she used the Woodcock–Johnson Tests of Achievement and the Gray Oral Reading Test

(psychological test from tests of academic performance). He was just at or below grade level in reading and above grade level in math.

- To evaluate his visual–spatial and motor functioning (processes underlying reading), she used the Rey–Osterrieth Complex Figure Test as well as the Beery Test of Visual Motor Integration. He was in the below average range.
- To assess his language performance (another process underlying learning) she used the Comprehensive Assessment of Spoken Language. He scored in the average range.
- To evaluate his general emotional development and functioning she used the Children's Apperception Test and the Kinetic Drawing System for School and Family (projective tests that require skilled interpretation). His stories in the CAT were often about a child being sad and disappointed in himself, and being teased by others.
- To assess specific categories of emotional difficulty, she asked David, his parents, and several of his teachers to complete the Conners' Attention Deficit Disorder Scales and the Achenbach Child Behavior Checklist (form questionnaires rating specific kinds of behavior). His score was high on the attention disorder scales and on the check list he was high on the internalizing scales (consistent with depression).

A few weeks later, after the psychologist reviewed and assessed the test results, she met with David and his parents to explain the specific findings and what they meant in terms of his learning and behavioral problems. She also summarized the findings in a written report that she gave to the family.

She said that David was an intelligent boy with good potential. He had enough problems with attentional and executive function to be diagnosed as having attention deficit disorder. She also thought that David had a specific learning disorder in processing written language and this showed up in problems with reading and writing. Both his problems with attention and language indicated reasons why he was not performing up to his potential.

He showed some emotional immaturity. He also had early signs of a mild reactive depression, which contributed to how quickly he felt incompetent and withdrew from a difficult task.

As part of an overall treatment program, the psychologist recommended further consultation with a child psychiatrist to evaluate David for the use of medication to help with his attention deficit disorder. She also gave specific recommendations to help his teachers work more effectively with him with regard to his reading and writing disorders, as well as his attentional problems. The teacher moved his seat to the front of the room to help him not be distracted by the activity of other children and to pay better attention to her.

She suggested parent counseling and individual psychotherapy for David, to help them all cope better with his attentional problems and his depression/low self-esteem difficulties.

* * *

Having read the chapter, you will be able to make more sense of whatever evaluation your child must undergo and of the information that the specialist gives you. Refer to this chapter when talking with your child's therapist, school staff, or psychiatrist (see Chapter 7 about helpers), who may make use of psychological or neuropsychological assessments to plan and carry out treatment (see Chapters 8, 9, and 10 on treatment).

Chapter 7

QUESTIONS ABOUT TREATMENT: WHO ARE THE HELPERS AND WHERE ARE THEY?

Once you decide to seek professional help for your child, you will encounter a confusing array of individuals who can provide consultation and treatment. The field of child mental health includes child psychiatrists, psychologists, social workers, family and marital therapists, counselors, and others. The goal of this chapter is to help you understand the different types of clinicians and the settings in which treatment is offered.

Organization of Chapter 7

I begin this chapter with some ideas to keep in mind as you seek and work with a professional. I then present information on the particular types of child mental health helpers. This information will include the following:

- their training and expertise
- what distinguishes one helper from another.

The information will help you find someone most suitable to your child's needs, have more realistic expectations of what any particular clinician can or cannot provide, and be better involved in your child's treatment.

I then explain the different settings where clinicians work. Knowing what distinguishes one setting from another can help you make sure that you are involved with the most appropriate resources for your child's problems. I specifically discuss outpatient care and the different levels of inpatient services, ranging from therapeutic schools to day hospitals to residential care.

Before you seek professional help

For many parents, the referral to a child specialist comes through a phone conversation with an agent of a managed care insurance company. Generally, the person making the referral does not know the particular professional to whom you and your child are being sent. Such a referral is not much more personal than if you had randomly looked up a specialist in the Yellow Pages of the telephone book. On the positive side, the insurance company must make sure that the individual they recommend has appropriate professional training and credentials.

If you are in a managed care program, I suggest that you first contact your pediatrician or family practitioner before calling your insurance plan to get a name. Your doctor will have had some contact with the professionals in your community and can give you better personal guidance. Generally, if you find a specialist on your own, the insurance company will not pay that professional unless he or she is already on the managed care insurance company's list, or "panel."

During the initial interview, you will talk about your child's difficulties *and* decide whether you want this clinician to work with your child. If, at the time of the first interview, you feel that you or your child are not a good match with a particular clinician, it is perfectly reasonable to interview someone else to find out if there might be a better fit. Of course, this freedom to choose the best fit may be narrow if the number of clinicians in your area is limited. For a discussion on other factors to keep in mind when seeking treatment, see Chapter 12, *Costs of Treatment: Money, Energy, and Time.*

Remember that mental health services are now more democratic and collaborative than in the past. You are encouraged to be involved in a professional's care of your child, so you need not wait "quietly" while the specialist is "figuring things out" and "making things better." Sharing your observations and concerns is *essential* to getting good treatment. Don't hesitate to ask questions:

- about your child's difficulties
- about your interaction with your child
- about someone else's interaction with your child
- about the clinician's understanding of your child and the treatment being offered.

If something is unclear to you or doesn't seem to be going in a direction that makes sense, ask. For example, if your child is on a medication that doesn't seem to be working, don't just stop the medication and not return to the doctor. Return and tell the doctor about your observations, doubts, and disappointments. You and your child's mental health specialist are trying to address complex matters. The better you can communicate with each other, the more likely you are to address the problem successfully.

Below, I describe eight types of professionals whom you may encounter on your path to getting help for your child. I start with the person you might begin with, your child's doctor, and then proceed roughly from the most to the least professionally trained child mental health specialist. These individuals are:

- pediatrician/family physician
- child psychiatrist
- clinical psychologist
- neuropsychologist
- clinical social worker
- family therapist
- mental health counselor
- school adjustment counselor.

For each professional, I describe their training, some distinguishing characteristics, and how to find that specialist.

Who are the helpers?

Pediatrician/family physician

This physician went to medical school and had three to five years' specialty training in the care of children or in family medicine. Your child's primary care doctor is a good place to start with your concerns, as your pediatrician or family physician is interested in your child's mind as well as body. Because some behavioral difficulties may be the outcome of a bodily medical disorder, it is good to get an evaluation and consultation with your child's doctor before seeing one of the other specialists below. Generally, pediatricians or family practitioners do not provide ongoing psychotherapy, although they may monitor and manage some of the medications used for treating emotional and behavioral difficulties. The pediatrician can help refer you to an appropriate child mental health clinician.

A *developmental pediatrician* is a pediatrician with two to three years' additional training that specializes in child development and behavior. This type of pediatrician spends much more time diagnosing and treating the complex developmental and behavioral disorders of childhood than general pediatric colleagues. Usually the developmental pediatrician is not involved in psychotherapy but gives recommendations and referrals for other kinds of treatment appropriate to your child's particular problem. This specialist will monitor and manage medications used to treat developmental and behavioral difficulties and often works with another child mental health clinician, like a clinical social worker or psychologist.

A *clinical nurse specialist* is a nurse trained in pediatrics and psychopharmacology. This individual frequently works along with a pediatrician or child psychiatrist and monitors a child's medications and overall mental condition. In some parts of the USA, clinical nurse specialists may have their own private practice.

Child psychiatrist

A child psychiatrist went to medical school and then had three or four years of general psychiatric training plus two more years of specialized child psychiatric training. Because of the training, this specialist has a comprehensive understanding of the developmental, medical/biological, psychological, and familial causes of the emotional and behavioral problems that occur in childhood. A child psychiatrist is the only child mental health specialist with training in childhood emotional and behavioral disorders who can provide talking therapy *and* prescribe medications. Since the 1980s medication treatment has become complicated and its use in children has increased. Thus nowadays a child psychiatrist may limit professional activity to evaluating a child, clarifying and identifying the problem, and prescribing medication. Some, however, still do both medication management and psychotherapy.

After evaluating and prescribing medication, the child psychiatrist may refer your child to a colleague to provide the psychotherapeutic treatment: a psychologist, social worker, or other licensed therapist. Typically, the psychiatrist will consult periodically with the therapist during the treatment.

In addition to asking your pediatrician or psychotherapist for a referral to a child psychiatrist, you can find this specialist under the listing "Physicians" in the Yellow Pages of the telephone book.

Unfortunately in the USA, there are fewer fully trained child psychiatrists than needed. In areas that have no child psychiatrist, a pediatrician, family practitioner, or general/adult psychiatrist prescribes medication and orders any medical tests, while a non-MD child professional provides psychotherapy.

Clinical psychologist

A clinical psychologist trained for three to five years post-college, earning either a master's or doctoral degree in psychology. The doctoral degree training is longer, more rigorous, and more advanced than the master's. If your child's problem is complicated, you might want the person with more training to treat him. A child psychologist has had further education in working with children, and is the only specialist who can both do sophisticated emotional and cognitive testing of your child *and* provide psychotherapy.

Not all clinical psychologists do both testing and therapy; some specialize in one or the other. The testing a psychologist does is used to help identify, explain, and guide treatment of your child's specific emotional, behavioral, and learning problems. (See Chapter 6 for more on psychological testing.) many psychologists work in schools.

Neuropsychologist

A neuropsychologist is a clinical psychologist with doctoral level training (PhD, EdD, PsyD) who has had some advanced training in the complex tests for cognitive/ learning disorders (see Chapter 6). Usually you would be referred to a neuropsychologist by your pediatrician/family practitioner, child psychiatrist, other mental health clinician, or school system staff. Neuropsychologists are listed under "Psychologists" in the Yellow Pages.

Clinical social worker

A clinical social worker trained for at least two years after college, learning how to provide talking therapy with individuals and families. He or she has expertise in psychological and psychosocial (groups and programs) treatments.

Sometimes people confuse the professional work of a clinical social worker with the work of a caseworker (sometimes also called a "social worker"). A caseworker usually works for a public social service agency and helps people manage the practical aspects of their lives. Typically, the caseworker has only a college degree or less, and not the more extensive formal training of a clinical social worker.

The majority of mental health specialists who have formal training in providing psychotherapy (in private practice or in clinics) are clinical social workers. Those who treat children have usually had some specialized formal training or additional work experience with children.

Clinical social workers who have completed a number of years of supervised practice and passed a licensing examination are called Licensed Independent Clinical Social Workers, or LICSW. Professional licensing and titles vary by state. Call your State Licensing Board to learn how the credentials of various mental health professionals are defined in your area.

Ordinarily you would be referred to a clinical social worker by a pediatrician or family practice doctor, child psychiatrist, or school counseling staff. You can find clinical social workers in private practice listed under the heading "Psychotherapists" or "Counseling" in the Yellow Pages.

Family therapist

Most individuals who do family therapy are clinical social workers. But some individuals get a single specialized degree in marital and family therapy. Such a person had two or more years in a post-college training program that focused on marriage and family therapy and is certified as a Licensed Marital and Family Therapist, or LMFT.

Any child's difficulties are inevitably entwined with how well a family is functioning. A child's difficulties may be a major stress upon the family, or the family difficulties may be a major stress upon the child. Helping a family function better almost always helps a child in distress.

A family therapist focuses on the family as a whole or on particular relationships within the family. Your pediatrician or family practice doctor, child psychiatrist, school counseling staff, or a clinician who works only with individuals (not with families) may refer you to a family therapist. You can find family clinicians under the heading "Psychotherapists" or "Counseling" in the Yellow Pages.

Mental health counselor

These individuals have master's level training in educational counseling (MEd) or psychological counseling (MA). They generally work in mental health clinics and are often called mental health counselors or technicians. They perform tasks similar to those of a clinical social worker or family therapist.

School adjustment counselor

School adjustment counselors may be trained as a guidance counselor, clinical social worker, or psychologist. Their work is confined to the school setting and academic year. They help students who are having emotional or behavioral problems in school that interfere with social or academic functioning. They may work with a child one-to-one or in a group.

A school adjustment counselor may refer your child to one of the above child mental health specialists outside the school. This will happen if the adjustment counselor thinks that your child's difficulties need more attention, time, or expertise than can be provided in the school setting alone.

The following table summarizes the types of professionals described above and includes which ones can prescribe medication, do testing, and provide individual or family therapy. It also describes where each type of professional works.

Table 7.1 Professionals: what they do and where they work

Professional	Does medical evaluations and can prescribe medication	Does complex psychological testing	Does individual child psychotherapy	Does family therapy	Works in mental health clinics and private office
Pediatrician	X				X (in *medical* settings)
Child psychiatrist	X		X	X	X
Child psychologist		X	X	X	X
Social worker			X	X	X
Family therapist				X	X

Where are the treatments?

Treatment is provided in either *outpatient* settings (clinics or private offices), *inpatient* settings (hospitals and residential programs), or *emergency* service settings (hospitals or clinics). Three factors determine which settings will be the location for treatment of your child:

- the intensity of the problem your child is having
- the complexity and duration of help needed to remedy the problem
- the availability or accessibility of services in your area.

Most child mental health treatment is done on an outpatient basis.

1. Outpatient services

Outpatient services generally take place in clinics (where multiple helpers work) or private offices (where a single individual works). Clinics might be private or public and are in settings such as a community mental health center, an outpatient department in a hospital, or an educational setting—from elementary school through college. In all settings, confidentiality is a priority. Three distinctions between clinics and private offices are worth noting:

- whether or not you know your helper before you receive treatment
- whether or not your helper has consultation from colleagues
- how the fees are determined.

In a clinic, generally you do not know who your helper will be before you go there. You and your child are assigned to a clinician who has an opening in her/his schedule. But most clinics let you switch to a different clinician if you and the assigned clinician are not working well together. By contrast, in a private office you will know in advance who you are going to see. And a bit more easily than in a clinic, you can switch to another practitioner if you do not think that you or your child will work well with that individual.

Clinics frequently provide clinicians with supervision, so there is ready access to consultation and collaboration about difficult situations. By contrast, a private practitioner may share and discuss complex clinical situations with a colleague but it is up to the individual to seek out consultation.

In the past, a clinic (public or private non-profit) was more likely to have a broader sliding fee scale than a private office practice. But managed care and a decrease in public funding have resulted in a much narrower sliding scale in non-profit clinics and in less of a difference from private practice (see Chapter 12 for more on costs of treatment).

The level of experience, competence, and investment in the work varies for individual professionals in both settings. Thus it is hard to say whether your treatment in a public clinic will be better than treatment in a private office.

Your pediatrician or family practitioner, child's school staff, managed care insurance company administrator, friends, or family members can help you find outpatient services.

2. Inpatient services

Inpatient services are usually provided in a hospital or a residential facility. I include therapeutic day school and day hospital treatment because even though your child still lives at home, these are intensive forms of treatment. Generally, intensive services are:

- tried *after* outpatient treatment
- undertaken because things seem to be getting worse
- viewed as very necessary to improve your child's condition.

Once inpatient services have helped your child enough so it seems safe and appropriate for him to return to family and community to receive outpatient treatment, he is discharged. Below, I describe these intensive services from the least to most intensive.

A. THERAPEUTIC DAY SCHOOL

If your child's main difficulty shows up in the regular school setting, a therapeutic day school is a good resource. Therapeutic day schools address school-related difficulties that are not simply academic but also involve emotional and behavioral problems. Generally, if a child cannot be adequately educated and behaviorally managed in a regular school setting, a therapeutic school is advised.

Therapeutic day school programs have more teachers per student than ordinary school settings; this gives adults more time and opportunity to work with a child's academic and emotional difficulties. Psychotherapeutic and psychopharmacological services typically are provided off the site of a therapeutic day school, elsewhere in the community, but occasionally some treatment services are provided right there.

Usually, the public school system helps to obtain and pay for a therapeutic day school program. You may encounter resistance from the administration of your child's school system when requesting a therapeutic day school because such services place a significant financial burden upon local communities. However, each state has laws requiring appropriate educational services to meet a child's needs. You may need the help of a child advocate to get the school system to respond with appropriate services.

B. DAY HOSPITAL/PARTIAL HOSPITALIZATION

If your child's difficulties are not seriously endangering enough to require hospitalization, he still may need more complex and intensive treatment than can be provided by just an ordinary outpatient setting. A day hospital program, if available, may be a logical alternative. In this type of program your child spends most of the day (often 8 a.m–4 p.m., occasionally evenings) involved in very intensive treatment but goes home at night to sleep. A day hospital program has a school component and a therapeutic component, which includes psychiatric medication monitoring and some combination of individual, group, and family therapies.

Your child might attend such a program for several weeks or a couple of months. Sometimes a day hospital program is used as a "step down" from a more intensive hospital setting or as a "step up" from a regular or therapeutic school program. The hope in using the day hospital as a "step up" is that a child can be intensively helped during a crisis or particularly difficult time and will, in a relatively short while, be able to return to the ongoing program. The cost of treatment is usually paid by insurance (public or private) and/or your child's public school system.

C. HOSPITAL

Generally, child psychiatric hospital services only are used for the most acutely endangered children. Your child needs a psychiatric hospital setting for treatment under the following conditions:

- if she is acutely suicidal or recurrently in jeopardy of causing serious self-harm
- if she is acutely homicidal or recurrently behaving aggressively and in jeopardy of seriously harming others
- if she experiences intensely disabling psychological symptoms.

During a hospital stay, your child will undergo diagnostic tests to eliminate treatable medical causes of her disordered emotions or behavior. She will probably receive medication, as well as intensive individual, family, and group treatment. The hospital staff seek to stabilize your child enough so that she can return to some form of treatment outside the hospital. It is in that post-hospital setting that less intensive, but longer-term, psychological and social forms of treatment are undertaken and medications monitored.

Hospital stays tend to be brief, in part because the daily cost is high. Since the cost is covered through insurance, either public or private, managed care companies aim to do everything they can to keep the length of the stay short. Representatives of the insurance company may have strong differences of opinion with the hospital staff about how long a child needs to be in the hospital setting for further treatment. Hospital stays also tend to be short because there are currently not enough child psychiatric inpatient services to meet the needs of children. So often, as soon as a child is doing better, she is quickly discharged to make room for a child doing poorly. Improvement with only a brief stay is possible largely because medication can have a positive effect quickly.

D. RESIDENTIAL TREATMENT

Treatment at a residential facility is the most comprehensive, complex, and long-term treatment available. Children usually stay in residential care for 6 to 18 months, sometimes longer. It is considered after other forms of treatment (outpatient, therapeutic school, day hospital, or hospital stay) have not succeeded. In certain situations, primarily those in which the home setting is thought to be a big factor in a child's difficulties, placement in a foster home or group home may be tried before residential treatment.

Your child may be placed in residential treatment if he seems at a chronic risk of seriously injuring himself or someone else. He may be unable to tolerate the stress of day-to-day life and be unmanageable by adults in school and at home. Most likely, professionals will consider placing your child in a residential facility if he has already been in a psychiatric hospital unit, often at least twice. Usually, the final decision on residential placement is made during a hospitalization; it may also be decided upon during a stay in a day-hospital program, an unsuccessful try at a therapeutic school, or during a course of outpatient treatment.

The components of residential care usually include 24-hour residential staffing, a therapeutic school, and on-site psychological and pharmacological/medication treatment. Psychological treatment usually includes individual, family, and group therapy. Residential staff provide supervision for the activities of daily living and for various on and off-grounds recreational activities. Residents may spend weekends at the facility or have home visits, depending upon how restrictive the program is and how close to home.

Usually residential care is paid for by both your child's school system and public agencies serving children's needs. Some states have one overriding agency to meet children's needs, for example the Department of Children's Services; others have the services separated out, such as the Department of Mental Health, Department of Mental Retardation, Department of Social Services, and Department of Youth Services. Like psychiatric hospitals for children, residential treatment facilities are expensive and in short supply.

3. Emergency/crisis services

For mental health emergencies, most communities use a local mental health crisis service or an emergency room at a local hospital. Generally the crisis service is staffed 24 hours a day, seven days a week.

Most child mental health emergencies involve a pressing threat of physical injury: either suicidal/self-destructive behavior or lethal/serious harm to others. Sometimes phone contact with staff members at an emergency service may be enough to address your child's crisis, particularly if the situation settles down when you call. However, face-to-face contact may be necessary. Most of the staff on emergency units are mental health technicians; some may be clinical social workers. Usually, a back-up psychiatrist is connected to the crisis service and can be contacted by the staff for consultation.

Respite beds for brief use may also be available at the crisis service. These are used as a way to avoid a hospitalization. Your child may stay in a respite bed instead of going to a hospital if:

- it looks like a day or two is enough time to defuse an explosive or dangerous situation

- managed care driven budgetary cuts and fiscal restraint dictate a brief stay in an emergency room rather than a more costly stay in a hospital

- there is no hospital bed available in your area at that time.

Generally, crisis staff are available to help through this interim period.

If your child is in ongoing treatment at the time of the crisis, the staff will usually notify your mental health clinician about the emergency event. In some cases that communication doesn't happen, so be sure to inform your mental health clinician any time that your child is involved with crisis or respite services.

* * *

This chapter's material has given you a background of who the specialists are, what they do or don't do, and what settings they work in. You are now ready to think about the specifics of the treatments that are offered. Chapter 8 on psychological treatments, Chapter 9 on medication treatments, Chapter 10 on alternative treatments, and Chapter 11 on the use of play in the treatment of children and adolescents give you such information.

Chapter 8

PSYCHOTHERAPY
AND ITS SIDE EFFECTS

After you decide to seek professional treatment for your child and find a mental health clinician to work with, you must evaluate the treatment being offered. This chapter, and Chapter 9, provide some basic information about the most commonly used treatments currently available.

There are two main categories of standard treatment: *psychological* (psychotherapy/talking therapy) and *psychopharmacological* (pharmacotherapy/medication). One may be undertaken without the other. However, each offers a different approach to problems. Therefore, especially with more difficult problems, psychological and pharmacological treatment might be used at the same time.

· If you choose to use the *complementary and alternative forms* of treatments (neurofeedback, meditation, sensory motor integration, vitamins and nutrition, herbal remedies) before, during, or after treatment with psychotherapy (Chapter 10), tell your child's clinician. If your child is going to be put on conventional medication in addition to psychotherapy, tell the prescribing doctor if your child is on any alternative medicinal, particularly any herbal remedy. There can be harmful consequences if certain conventional and alternative chemical treatments are combined.

Organization of Chapter 8

In this chapter I do the following:

1. Provide an overview of psychological treatments and their side effects.

2. Address seven common questions that arise for parents about psychological treatment, including:

   • What type of child mental health specialist might be best to provide psychological treatment?

   • Which form of psychological treatment might be most helpful?

- What is considered when trying to judge how effective the treatment is and how long to continue?

- What is considered when trying to decide about using medication and psychological treatment together?

Psychological treatment

Psychotherapy/psychotherapeutic help is a form of treatment for emotional and behavioral difficulties that depends entirely upon talking; in other words, it is psychological treatment. Many different kinds of psychotherapy exist. Each varies in terms of both what the client talks about and how he or she talks about it. Some forms of psychotherapy rely more heavily upon specific educational techniques, such as practicing certain behaviors or having homework. Other forms are more personal and rely more heavily upon the development of a relationship between the client and therapist. (Chapter 11 describes in more detail how and why psychotherapeutic treatment works.) Most psychotherapy, even types that are more educational, require some form of a relationship to be effective.

Psychotherapy is more democratic and collaborative than in the past. To make the treatment successful, your and your child's questions, concerns, observations, and reactions to the therapy itself are important ingredients. This shift parallels wider societal changes in health care relationships that now place less emphasis on a professional's authority for decisions and more on informed patients sharing in decisions. This more democratic approach also comes from an understanding that collaboration leads to better and more long-lasting constructive change.

Each type of psychotherapy can differ not only in the focus and content but also in the degree of knowledge, sophistication, and expertise with which it is carried out by a professional. See the "Frequently asked questions" at the end of this chapter for more about expertise. Below, I describe individual psychotherapy generally, and the most common forms.

Individual psychotherapy

Individual psychotherapy involves your child or adolescent meeting alone with a mental health specialist (psychotherapist) for 30 to 50 minutes, typically once per week. Often the parent has a separate regular meeting with the therapist; this is less common if the patient is an adolescent. Table 8.1 provides overviews of the main forms of individual psychotherapy.

COGNITIVE BEHAVIORAL THERAPY (CBT)

CBT is structured, directive, and homework is frequently assigned. The therapist will work with your child primarily on her thoughts and behaviors.

Table 8.1 Characteristics of the main forms of individual psychotherapy

Types of individual psychotherapy	Process of change: mainly through education or through the relationship	Main topic of the talk	Focus of the talk: mainly directed (by therapist) or non-directed (chosen by client/patient)	Approximate treatment length
Cognitive behavioral therapy (CBT)	Education	Thoughts and behaviors	Directed	1–3 months
Dialectical behavior therapy (DBT)	Education	Emotions, thoughts, behaviors, and present relationships	Directed	1 year +/–
Psychodynamic psychotherapy	Relationship	Emotions, thoughts, and past and present relationships	Non-directed	Few months to a few years
Interpersonal psychotherapy (ITP)	Education and relationship	Emotions, thoughts, and present relationships	Directed to main topic, but then non-directed	3–4 months
Eye movement desensitization and reprocessing (EMDR)	Education (technique)	Specific traumatic memories (images and thoughts)	Directed to images/thoughts and alternates with non-directed talk	3–12 sessions
Psychoanalysis	Relationship	Emotions, thoughts, and past and present relationships	Non-directed	4–5 times a week for one to several years

A central assumption of this approach is that the thoughts, feelings, and behaviors that are "the problem" must be distinguished from your child's underlying patterns and habitual ways of thinking and behaving. For example, suppose your child is actively avoiding some particular place, person, or circumstance, and reporting she "just doesn't like" what she is avoiding. Probably her avoidant behavior is caused by deeper frightening feelings, images, and thoughts that come up when she approaches a feared situation. CBT helps your child become more aware of her underlying irrational thoughts that are present when intense fear or anxiety are present.

Identifying and talking about those thoughts decreases their intensity and the likelihood of acting on them. The therapist will help your child challenge the irrational underlying thoughts by encouraging her to practice new behavioral patterns. Taking actions contrary to those illogical thinking patterns adds an important step towards changing the thinking and its connected behavior. This is why the therapist helps your child actively confront, engage, and face what she has been avoiding.

For example, your child might very much want to have a sleep-over at a friend's house, but has to be picked up early because he becomes too frightened and panicked as the night wears on. As a younger child he may have been a bedwetter and had a shaming experience at the house of a friend. Although it may have been several years since the bedwetting and shaming incident, his worry may have grown quite large. With a CBT therapist, your son would draw up a list of potentially embarrassing situations and circumstances, each increasingly stressful. They would explore the irrational elements in each situation. Your son would also learn that being embarrassed was a normal human experience and did not mean that he was a failure. Then he would actively confront his fear by tackling each situation. He would start with the easiest one first and work his way to the hardest: first having friends over to his house, then sleeping over at a friend's house nearby, and finally having a sleep-over with a friend across town.

Research has found that CBT helps adults for depression, phobias, panic attacks, and compulsions. Recent research indicates that it is also helpful for children. It may be difficult to find therapists who consider themselves specialists in CBT, but many therapists use cognitive behavioral techniques and interventions in their work.

DIALECTICAL BEHAVIORAL THERAPY (DBT)

DBT is an expanded form of cognitive behavioral treatment that involves coordinated work in individual psychotherapy and in group therapy. DBT is perhaps best known for its group component called "skills training" (see group treatment, below).

In individual psychotherapeutic work, DBT focuses on a recent incident of problem behavior. The goal is to understand the triggers and causes of the behavior. The therapist and client look at the emotional, cognitive (ways of thinking), and social factors involved. Once the child gains understanding of those factors, she and the therapist focus on developing better responses to the specific triggers.

Learning to manage emotions, particularly anger, is central to DBT. For example, if your daughter were to engage in self-cutting behavior, the therapist and she would try to understand what happened that led up to the behavior. They would identify the events preceding it and the thoughts and emotions present before, during, and after the events, as well as before and during the cutting. Then the focus would shift to different ways of thinking about the triggering events and of dealing with the emotions that came up.

Usually the work involves the child practicing specific skills or techniques to improve modulating and balancing emotions, coping with distress, managing interpersonal relations, and improved self-awareness. In DBT more attention is given to the therapeutic relationship than in conventional CBT. The therapist tries to balance validating/accepting the patient's current emotional experience and working towards behavioral change.

So the therapist might validate the intensity of her emotional distress, acknowledge that the cutting behavior was an attempt to cope with that pain, but remind her that they were working together to help her find better ways to cope with her distress that would eventually take the place of the cutting.

Individual DBT, along with the skills group component, has been shown to help individuals whose lives are filled with emotional turmoil as well as interpersonal and psychological crises. For example, DBT has been used with adults with a history of physical or sexual trauma and self-injurious/suicidal actions. Recently, it has been used increasingly with adolescents who have self-injurious or suicidal behavior, or who struggle with troubling behaviors (such as substance abuse and eating disorders) or with tumultuous emotions (such as severe mood disorders and intense anxiety).

PSYCHODYNAMIC PSYCHOTHERAPY

Psychodynamic psychotherapy focuses primarily on your child's feelings and thoughts about himself and others, particularly as they surface in important relationships with family and friends. Usually, when someone just uses the term "psychotherapy" alone, they are referring to psychodynamic psychotherapy. With children and adolescents, when appropriate, psychodynamic psychotherapy often involves the use of play. Your child's therapist, whether using specific play therapy techniques (see Chapter 11) or not, tries to understand your child's deeper emotional experience. The therapist then communicates this understanding to your child during their work together. Two goals of this process are to help your child find better ways to cope with feelings and to develop a better ability to distinguish between how he feels about an event and the event itself. Improving these two abilities will positively affect your child's self-image and his behavior with others. See Chapter 11 for more about this kind of therapy.

While psychodynamic psychotherapy may focus on particular symptoms, this treatment is not as symptom-focused as CBT. For example, your child may be experiencing a great deal of anxiety and depression a few months following the unexpected death of his teacher. The focus of psychodynamic work may not be as much on the specific symptoms (such as fear of being alone or obsessive worries) that led him to come to therapy as it might be on what emotions (fear, sadness, and guilt) remained unsettled from that event, what may be contributing to the unsettledness, and what he needs to better resolve the emotions from that experience.

INTERPERSONAL PSYCHOTHERAPY (ITP)

ITP is psychodynamic psychotherapy that is more focused and time-limited (12–16 sessions). This treatment focuses on specific difficulties that led your child to be in therapy, such as:

- unresolved loss/grief
- changes in life roles (starting a new school, living with a new step-parent)
- conflict with a particular person
- problems getting along with others in general.

ITP is more suitable for adolescents than younger children because the focused and time-limited nature of the work uses less play and more language than open-ended psychodynamic psychotherapy.

EYE MOVEMENT DESENSITIZATION AND REPROCESSING (EMDR)

EMDR may refer to an eight-phase form of individual psychotherapy, originally developed to address traumatic memories, or to a technique for improving the processing of disturbing memories or images. A trained clinician can incorporate the technique into various forms of individual psychotherapy. In simplified form, it involves having the patient pay simultaneous attention to an internal traumatic memory (image or thought) and to a moving external image (the therapist's finger) that the therapist moves back and forth so that the patient's eyes cross the midline from side to side. Primarily developed and used for treating trauma-related symptoms in adults, it has increasingly been used for other types of adult symptoms and with children and adolescents who have trauma-related symptoms.

PSYCHOANALYSIS

Psychoanalysis is a specialized form of psychodynamic psychotherapy that allows more time to focus on unconscious patterns of thought and feeling. It is very intensive (meetings four to five times per week for two or more years). Typically, psychoanalysis is used when other forms of psychological treatment have not been sufficiently helpful.

PARENT COUNSELING

Parent counseling involves the child's therapist meeting with the parents without the child. It is not a form of individual psychotherapy but is usually done along with it.

Individual therapy for school-aged children should always be accompanied by parent counseling. Parents may meet with a therapist even if individual therapy is not ordinarily undertaken (as with a very young child). This might also happen if individual therapy is not possible (as with an adolescent refusing individual treatment).

The focus of parent counseling is upon the parent–child interaction, not the marital situation, unless it is specified as a focus of the work. The goal is to help you, the parent, better understand your child and learn better ways of dealing with particular situations involving your child.

For parents of adolescents, parent counseling probably is best done in family therapy or by a different therapist from the person treating the adolescent. But sometimes such options are not practically possible, so the adolescent therapist may provide occasional parent counseling sessions.

The therapist may have a brief contact with you at the beginning or end of your child's session. This is *not* parent counseling. This is only for brief communication and does not give enough time to engage thoughtfully around particular parent–child matters.

Non-individual psychotherapy

Non-individual therapy involves people in addition to just your child and therapist, in some kind of group. Your child learns through hearing others' perspectives, experiences, and struggles, as well as through the interactions that take place within the group during the meetings. The therapist may encourage and observe the group members' interactions, actively participate in the interactions, or some combination of these two roles.

Usually non-individual psychotherapy complements individual therapy, although sometimes it may be the only type of treatment indicated or available. Family or group therapy as part of the treatment for a younger child can be done by the same therapist who does individual therapy.

FAMILY THERAPY

Family therapy focuses mainly on the interactions between parents and children. The goals are to help the family as a whole, and various members of the family, communicate, understand, and function better with one another.

Family therapy can be done in many ways, based on different theoretical perspectives. Typically, meetings occur weekly and last for 50 minutes or longer.

Sessions may include other family members in addition to just the parents and the child whose symptoms triggered treatment. Some family therapists may:

- include everyone who is living in the household
- include any significant family members who live close by and are actively involved with the family
- meet with different subunits of the family, for example only with siblings, or with just one parent and the child identified as the "patient."

Individual therapy may not be a possibility with your child or adolescent because of his strong opposition to acknowledging or focusing on his difficulties. In that case, the choice of family therapy, and focusing upon difficulties between family members, may be more acceptable and ultimately more helpful.

choice of family therapy, and focusing upon difficulties between family members, may be more acceptable and ultimately more helpful.

GROUP THERAPY

Group therapy involves your child or adolescent meeting with peers who may share similar difficulties. Group therapy may be a mix of action and talking (as in play therapy with younger children), or may be mostly talking (for teenagers).

Group therapy aims to help your child/adolescent develop better social skills and/or a better understanding and ability to cope with particular problems or situations. Your child may find it easier to learn about his behavior from peers than from adults. The safety developed in ongoing group therapy can help him tolerate insights and self-awareness that are painful but beneficial.

Generally, a single group session lasts about 90 minutes. Groups tend to have a preset time frame: they may last the school year, or four to six months. If your child still needs more group therapy when that time frame ends, he may join the next group that forms.

DBT SKILLS GROUP TRAINING

DBT (dialectical behavioral therapy) skills group training is a form of group therapy that focuses on learning, reviewing, and practicing specific social and self-management skills. The material is presented in a particular structure and format, in four modules:

- mindfulness
- distress tolerance
- interpersonal effectiveness
- emotional regulation.

This type of group is often ongoing: participants leave the group after completing one or more cycles of the four modules. As old members leave, new participants enter.

This approach has been so helpful in clinics and private practice that counselors have now begun to use a modified form of skills training in schools.

Choosing a therapist

If you are not familiar with the field of psychotherapy, choosing a therapist and a form of therapy for your child may feel like a blind act of faith. When choosing, keep these guidelines in mind:

- Try to have the therapist *recommended* to you, by your pediatrician or some other trustworthy resource, as someone who is knowledgeable and professional.

- Before you make your final decision, meet with the therapist and feel comfortable that this person will understand you and your concerns.

- Seek an individual with whom you believe your child will feel safe and at ease.

In the next section, I address common questions about various aspects of psychotherapy for your child. My answers will help you understand psychotherapy and be a more informed participant in the treatment.

Psychotherapy: frequently asked questions

1. DOES IT MATTER WHETHER THE THERAPIST IS AN MD, PHD, MSW OR OTHER TRAINED PERSON?

The short answer is "no." What matters most is how much experience and practice the therapist has in child psychotherapy.

Having said this, generally you do want the person who is most highly trained to work with your child, since it is assumed that the more advanced the training, the better the treatment. But you cannot tell, just based on a therapist's degree, how experienced in child psychotherapy an individual is. A child psychiatrist may know a lot *about* child psychotherapy. But since the field has begun to emphasize medication, many child psychiatrists spend more time prescribing medicine than actually doing child psychotherapy.

Ideally you want someone who has had advanced training that draws upon the wisdom of experts in the field *and* has had experience doing such treatment with children. These days, most child psychotherapy is done by individuals with an MSW (Masters in Social Work: see Chapter 7). Typically, MSWs have had supervised training in treating children psychologically and have gained skill through ongoing experience.

In complex situations that require both medication and psychotherapy, it is best to have one person do both. But that is often hard to do since few child psychiatrists also do psychotherapy.

Remember, too, that just because an individual has good professional training and experience does not guarantee that he or she will form a good alliance with your particular child (see Question 3 below).

2. WHAT FACTORS MAY AFFECT WHICH FORM OF THERAPY WILL BE PROVIDED TO MY CHILD?

The training of the therapist

Whether the clinician is in a clinic or a private office in the larger community, the training of that person will determine which type of therapy you receive. If a particular therapist only does individual therapy or only family therapy, then that is the therapy you will be offered. The same is true if a particular individual therapist does only CBT or only psychodynamic play therapy. Fortunately, there is overlap in the effectiveness of these different treatments, so skilled clinicians providing different forms of treatment can be similarly helpful.

The age of your child

Usually children under ages seven to eight are best served by psychodynamic play therapy, since they have a limited ability to verbalize and reflect on their experience. As your child gets older, there is more of a choice to be made between therapy that is more cognitive behavioral and therapy that is more psychodynamic. Group therapy and family therapy also become more possible as your child gets older. Individual therapy for school-aged children, those who are not yet adolescents, should always be accompanied by parent counseling. Sometimes parent counseling alone, without individual therapy for a younger child, may be the best course to follow.

While the individual therapist for a younger child is usually the same person who provides parent counseling, this is more complicated with an adolescent. Most teens want their confidentiality and autonomy respected. Therefore some individual therapists will not meet with the parents of an adolescent without the adolescent being present, and if they do, they will tell the teen in detail what the conversation was about.

Many therapists find that doing individual therapy and family therapy with the same teen is too complex. Therefore they recommend that one therapist provides individual therapy and a different therapist provides family therapy. But some therapists will do both, since they think this has more benefits than drawbacks. In making these decisions, the adolescent's maturity level is even more important than his chronological age.

The severity of the problem

Sometimes, as when a child is having a severe problem at home and with others, it is clear from the start that one particular psychotherapeutic approach is not going to work. Sometimes it is clear that a combination of two forms of psychotherapy (such as individual and family therapy) is needed. The therapist should be able to explain to you why he or she recommends a combination, so that the time, effort, and cost for such an undertaking make sense.

Parental resources: finances, time, and energy

Taking a child to individual therapy once a week, and having parental counseling or family therapy weekly or every other week, consumes time, energy, and money. This is even more so if family therapy or individual treatment for the parent is indicated; it can seem as if time is totally taken up with therapy and transportation to and from therapy.

For parents with insurance and limited personal financial resources, the decision about which therapist may be seen is made largely by the managed care insurance company. Even parents with more resources must decide how much money, time, and energy is to be spent on treatment for a particular child, or for themselves, and how much for other family members and other needs. Discuss such dilemmas with the therapist. And remember that usually psychotherapy is a time-limited demand.

3. HOW DO I JUDGE WHETHER OR NOT PSYCHOTHERAPY IS HELPING MY CHILD?

The best way to know if therapy is helping is to see whether or not your child's behavior or internal state has improved. Usually you would see this change within four to six months.

But during the early stages of psychotherapy and of improvement, it might not be so clear whether the psychotherapy is effective. Early signs that therapy is working may include the following:

- your child or adolescent seems more willing to go to psychotherapy
- your child's problematic behavior or emotions decrease in intensity or frequency
- your child has an increase in more positive behaviors and emotional states.

If within four to six months you do not see change outside of therapy, bring this observation up with your child's therapist. It may be that the form of therapy offered is insufficient for the problem. After discussion with the therapist, you may decide to add another form of therapy, such as family or group therapy, to the individual therapy (see Question 5 below for a discussion about adding *medications* to psychotherapy).

4. WHAT IF WE ARE THINKING ABOUT SWITCHING THERAPISTS?

If therapy does not seem to be helping, you may find yourself thinking about switching therapists. Do not do this abruptly. Instead, raise your concerns, observations, doubts, and questions about the treatment. If the therapist is open to addressing these matters, that means you are working together to figure out the best course. If the therapist does *not* respond to your concerns, however, or seems not to respect you when you bring up such matters, your clinician is not working with you and you should then switch therapists.

5. HOW LONG WILL THE PSYCHOTHERAPY LAST?

Focused psychotherapy (such as CBT, interpersonal psychotherapy, or short-term psychodynamic psychotherapy or family therapy) will usually take place within a two to five-month time frame.

Longer-term psychodynamic psychotherapy and play therapy may last from six to eighteen months or more. Treatment is provided continuously over that time. Depending upon the therapist's training, the severity of the problem, and resources available, the sessions might be one, two, or more times per week. Family therapy (commonly one time per week) may last for six months, and usually more.

Sometimes therapy may take place in blocks or phases. Treatment may end with the understanding that the child may return later for further therapy. This could be recommended if some problems that have been identified still remain and cannot at that time be sufficiently addressed. Or, returning later may make sense if the therapist expects new problems are likely to arise, but cannot treat these problems "preventatively."

6. HOW MUCH OF WHAT GOES ON IN PSYCHOTHERAPY WITH MY CHILD WILL I BE TOLD?

Regardless of the child's age, a therapist will generally share information that comes up in treatment if a child's safety is endangered. In terms of information that does not impact on safety, the therapist will treat the matter for younger children and adolescents differently.

Children up to fifth grade pretty much expect that the parent is privy to all that goes on within the playroom, although the therapist will use his or her discretion with that expectation. Older children, particularly adolescents, take confidentiality seriously. A therapist who is trying to develop a working relationship with an adolescent must diligently protect confidentiality and only break it when seriously worried about life-threatening circumstances.

It is usually not helpful, for the parent or for the child/adolescent patient, if the parent knows details about what is going on within the individual therapy. But you may certainly ask the therapist for a general understanding of what is happening in the treatment. Questions about your child's therapy may come up for many reasons. Raise such questions with the therapist, particularly when it may be your first experience with child mental health treatment.

7. HOW DO I DECIDE WHETHER TO HAVE MY CHILD TAKE MEDICATION IN ADDITION TO, OR INSTEAD OF, PSYCHOTHERAPY?

In Chapter 9, I discuss the question about when it is appropriate to add psychotherapy to treatment with medications. Here I discuss when it is appropriate to add *medication* to psychological treatment.

When pharmacological treatment first began to be used with adults, psychotherapists thought that medication would undermine engagement in psychotherapy. But later, therapists found that for many people, medication allowed the psychotherapy to go deeper and to be more effective. That has also been found to be true for children and adolescents.

If your child is too depressed, anxious, agitated, or guarded, she may not be able to engage with the therapist in a way that makes the psychotherapy useful. In that case, she may not improve much, and her behavioral and emotional difficulties can persist or even get worse, despite psychotherapy. In such circumstances, medication may give your child a better chance to engage with the therapist and gain from psychotherapy.

Sometimes psychotherapy is agonizing for a child; symptoms don't respond to the treatment and medication is started. After going on medication, a child may continue to skip appointments, refuse to go, or sit silently throughout every session, while outside the therapy he improves. If that happens with your child, do *not* just drop out of psychological treatment and continue only with medication. Instead, consult with the psychotherapist and the doctor providing medication and try to get a better grasp of what is going on (see Questions 3 and 4 above). Remember: psychological treatment and pharmacological treatment each provide something that the other form of treatment does not.

Psychotherapy and side effects

It may seem strange to talk about side effects from psychotherapy. However, just as there are unwanted or unexpected consequences (beneficial or detrimental) to the use of medication, so too are there to psychotherapy. The following are five types of side effects that come up in psychotherapy.

1. Sometimes, early in treatment, your child may actually have a brief increase in symptoms. This is especially likely with the more exploratory, psychodynamic type of psychotherapy. Your child's increase in anger or sadness may be associated with the pressure or turbulence from thoughts and feelings that, up until that time, she has managed largely by avoiding or suppressing them. Early in treatment, your child may not trust the therapist enough to contain the pressure of these emotions. If your child seems more anxious or oppositional after a few sessions, this state of increased anxiety generally will pass as treatment moves along. Explain this to your child.

2. Your child's emotional distress may also increase after she's been in treatment for a while. This can happen when a particularly stressful stage in the psychotherapy has been reached and disturbing thoughts, feelings, and memories come up. Her distress may show up as resistance to attending sessions or an increased irritability, or sadness, at home. When you suspect there are side effects, consult with the treating clinician. Air your concerns that therapy is not going well. Tell the therapist about some difficulty your child is having with the therapy that may not show up so clearly within the sessions.

3. Your teen, or occasionally a younger child, may inadvertently create or expose misunderstanding and conflict between parents and therapist. She may bring up something that the therapist allegedly said which seems provocative and insensitive. This could happen because:

    • the therapist may have said something that was unprofessional

    • your child may be misinterpreting what was said

    • your child might be reporting the incident in a distorted way because she is testing your motivation for the treatment and support of the therapist

    • it's your child's way of expressing her desire to get out of going to therapy.

In such circumstances, you may find yourself feeling confused and being drawn into the therapy in a way that feels uncomfortable and negative. You may find it helpful to talk more with your child about her feelings concerning the therapist's statement. Then, if appropriate, you might decide to take a "wait and see" approach. Or, after asking your child's or adolescent's permission, you may want to speak directly with the therapist about the matter.

4. Psychotherapy may be aimed not only at helping a child better adapt to circumstances, but also at fostering freedom of expression, maturity, and autonomy. Usually parents welcome this change in their child. But sometimes, your child's increased self-assertiveness may be unsettling for you, since it challenges your own perspective and authority. Because such challenges were not there before therapy, parents may view such behavior as an unwanted "side effect."

5. Finally, a child may find the therapeutic setting and therapist so supportive and helpful that she may become excessively dependent on or attached to the therapist for a while. It may be irritating to family members if the child frequently talks about the therapist and what the therapist says. Such behavior may be due to your child's dealing with difficult emotions like anxiety or shame through idealizing the therapist. This response may be a "side effect" of becoming more involved in the psychotherapy. The response is often short-lived, especially when addressed within the therapy.

* * *

I hope that the material in this chapter increases the likelihood that you and your child will experience the benefits of psychotherapy. It can be an extremely helpful way to get "back on track" for you and your child. It also might be an eye-opening experience that positively affects unexpected aspects of your lives. For some, it is only frustrating and disappointing. For more detail about psychotherapy, and play therapy in particular, see Chapter 11.

Chapter 9

MEDICATIONS AND THEIR SIDE EFFECTS

This chapter will give you some basic information and understanding of medications currently used to treat children.

The use of medication to improve emotional or behavioral symptoms is called *psychopharmacological treatment*, or *pharmacotherapy*. Usually the symptoms addressed are severe enough to interfere with normal daily functioning or are very distressing to your child.

As I said in Chapter 8, there are two main categories of conventional treatment: *psychological* (psychotherapy/talking therapy) and *psychopharmacological* (pharmacotherapy/medication). Each may be undertaken without the other. But since each provides something the other does not, treatment of more distressing or hard to resolve problems often involves the simultaneous use of psychological and pharmacological therapies.

In this chapter, almost all of the medications I describe are *synthesized*: they do not occur naturally. For information about naturally occurring chemicals used in treatment refer to the discussion of alternative treatments in Chapter 10. Tell the doctor who will be prescribing medication for your child whether or not she/he is already on any alternative medicinal, particularly herbal, remedy. There can be harmful consequences if certain conventional and alternative chemical treatments are combined (see Chapter 10, "Herbal treatment").

Organization of Chapter 9

The first section of this chapter addresses three topics:

- how medications/chemicals affect behavior
- general guidelines for using medication with children
- side effects in general, and particularly with regard to medication.

I then discuss medications that are used for five categories of symptoms:

- inattention, impulsivity, hyperactivity, and distractibility
- depression
- bipolar disorder and severe mood instability
- anxiety
- psychosis (schizophrenia, paranoia), and severe symptoms of mood, anxiety, aggression, and agitation.

For each category, I describe the kinds of medications used and explain common and concerning side effects. I encourage you to skim the material concerning the five categories of symptoms for the specific information you need on the medications your child is taking, or may take, to address his particular symptoms.

At the end of the chapter, I explore some of the common questions and issues about medication treatment that crop up for parents. Topics include:

- Who is the best person to provide medication treatment for your child, and why?
- How do you decide to have your child take medication? Should your child take medication with, or instead of, psychotherapy?
- How do you tell whether medication is helping?
- How long will pharmacotherapy last?
- Will pharmacotherapy continue without psychotherapy?

How medications/chemicals affect behavior

We currently understand that medications change the balance and concentration of specific chemicals in the brain, like serotonin, norepinephrine and dopamine. These natural brain chemicals play important roles in how we think, feel, pay attention, and behave. But we still do not know very much of the details about how or why medications can be as helpful as they are.

How, then, can you both make sense of the way medications help with your child's complex emotional and behavioral problems and also communicate this understanding clearly to your child?

Basically, medications help your child to *modulate*, or keep in balance, his or her emotions, thoughts, attention, or behavior. Medications help achieve this balance in two ways:

- by toning down the intensity of disruptive emotions and highly emotional thoughts
- by improving the screening out of distracting stimulation.

Your child's improved balance may show up in his emotions, thoughts, attention, behavior, or all four. That improved balance will help your child use his best developed *coping skills* to deal with ordinary and stressful situations. "Best coping skills" means, for example, that your child can slow down an impulse to act and consider the best way to react to a situation or ask for an adult's help in a difficult situation. Or your child might be able to use language as a way to address a problem (rather than acting on it physically) or to tolerate a certain degree of emotional discomfort that is naturally part of a situation (rather than immediately becoming belligerent or fleeing). When your child uses his best coping skills, he is better at communicating with others, understanding the world, and modulating, tolerating, and appreciating his own inner experience. Medications may help with almost any intense symptom that prevents your child from using his best developed coping skills.

This view of medication as helping your child keep balance encourages your child to take a more active role towards helping himself get "back on track." Your child, instead of seeing the medicine as something that "makes me" behave or feel better, more likely will think of the medication as something that "helps me" behave or feel better. He is less likely to feel like a passive recipient of his emotional and behavioral life.

General guidelines for using medication with children

Parents and other adults often ask me, "How can the doctor make a decision about using medication for my child after only seeing us for just 15, 30, or 45 minutes?" This is a good question.

Such brief evaluations do a disservice to the individual complexity of a child and do not help foster a strong working partnership. However, after considering any existing medical problems and allergic sensitivities, it is fairly straightforward to match medications to symptoms, as each type of symptom may be helped with one of several medications. At our present state of knowledge, it does not generally seem to matter much what age or gender your child is, or what the psychological cause of the symptoms may be. Medications help in a way that is unrelated to the particular circumstances or situation.

It is hard to give specific guidelines for all instances of pharmacotherapy. Each child is unique, each problem situation is somewhat different, and there are many kinds of medications to choose from. However, several general principles can guide medication usage in children.

1. *Medication is used to address the severity of symptoms more than the presence of symptoms.* Medication is not automatically prescribed simply because a child experiences depressive symptoms, anxiety, or attentional problems. The use of medication will depend upon how severe the symptom is: how disruptive and how painful, and how responsive to psychotherapy and

other interventions it has been. The severity of a symptom is a guide when assessing the balance of potential benefits and risks from the use of medication (see guideline 5). Milder symptoms may represent a stage in growing up and are better handled by coping with the particular task in development than by removing the symptom.

2. *After a symptom has diminished greatly or disappeared for six to twelve months, it is reasonable to lower the medication gradually to discover how much, if any, is still needed.* A gradual reduction works best because reactions to lowering the medication are less likely than if it is dropped or stopped suddenly. If symptoms do return at the lower dose, they are usually less intense and more easily managed, and the dose can be put back to the higher level. This principle of slowly lowering the medication is simply the reverse direction of the way medication is often begun: at a low dose and slowly increased to an optimal amount.

3. *More than one medication may be prescribed at a time, but it is best to* change *only one medication at a time.* Your child may be on more than one medication if one medication doesn't help quite enough and another is needed, or if a second medication is used to reduce the side effects caused by the first medication. If a child is on two or more medications yet is still not well enough, the doctor may consider a change. It isn't always clear which medication is helpful. When trying to figure this out, change just one medication at a time. This increases the chance of figuring out which medication is helpful.

4. *Most psychotropic medications currently used with children have no apparent long-term harmful medical effects.* I say "apparent" because most medications used in children have not been studied for long enough to make the statement definitively. There is no evidence of increased abnormal development or increases in serious diseases like cancer or neurological disorders. However, we do know that *some* medications can cause serious side effects (short and long term). A child should be monitored for the development of these side effects (see discussion of side effects below).

5. *The use of medication for any particular child always involves a judgment about the unknown.* There are possible side effects of using medication. There also are probable effects of not using medication: your child will continue to suffer. In my experience, using medication for a child who is in severe emotional and behavioral distress more often leads to *less* harmful outcomes than not using medication. A child in severe distress may engage in impulsive actions aimed at relieving emotional pain but which often lead to more harm and more problems. Proper treatment sometimes can keep that from happening.

6. *A child should be actively engaged in his own medication treatment.* This includes participating in the decision to use medication and evaluating whether or not the medication is working. This is particularly so for an adolescent who is at a stage in life that involves taking on more self-responsibility and independence.

7. *The doctor should fully explain the reason for the use of a particular medication.* Knowing why a particular medicine is prescribed and how it is supposed to help can lessen resistance to taking medication. The doctor and parent ought to help a child understand:

   • the name of the medication being taken

   • the reason for taking it

   • how the medication is supposed to help

   • what the dosage is.

Information about medications can be hard to understand. In the next section, I give an overview of side effects in general and medications in particular. This should help you make better sense of the medication options for particular symptoms, and their potential benefits and risks, which I provide later in the chapter.

Side effects in general

The term side effect refers to the *unintended consequences* that may go along with a treatment. This term is used most frequently when talking about medication. But other forms of treatment in medicine—such as surgery, radiation treatment, physical therapy—also have unintended consequences. Occasionally, unintended consequences may have positive benefits. But usually, the unwanted, negative consequences are our greatest concern. This is why doctors take the long-standing Hippocratic Oath, "First, do no harm."

Our lives are always filled with many actual and potential "unintended consequences." The common term for such unintended and unwanted consequences is "bad luck." Generally, the more complex the action, the more likely are such unintended consequences.

Sometimes, because we know that complex actions—including taking psychotropic drugs—can lead to unintended and unwanted consequences, we mistakenly think that such actions should never be taken. This is a *risk-avoidant response*, driven by worry.

The opposite response, called the *risk denial response*, is also driven by worry. This view proposes that since there may be unintended consequences for any action, you simply should move ahead, do whatever a doctor suggests, and "don't think about it." This view leads people to make decisions without enough information, and prevents people from taking the necessary steps to minimize the likelihood of side effects.

I encourage a middle path. Be clear about what the benefits of a medication are for your child and be aware of the possible side effects. Remember, "doing nothing" is nevertheless an action. The sources for your child's disorder, disruption, or pain are always changing. If you take no action, the problem could get better on its own, but it could become worse and more intense.

If you take this middle position, you will have to learn to tolerate uncertainty while making a decision. Frequently, it is hard to decide whether "action" (taking medication or entering into psychotherapy) or "no action" (not taking those steps) more likely will lead to better benefits and fewer negative, unintended consequences.

Medications in children and side effects

Side effects may occur with any medicine: conventional or alternative. Parents may find that reading the list of possible side effects for a given medication is quite daunting. But remember the following:

- Many children taking medication have no side effects at all.

- Even common side effects do not occur in everyone.

- Common side effects generally do not occur in the majority of patients taking the medication.

- More serious side effects are best dealt with by knowing about their possibility and planning with the doctor the most appropriate action at the first sign of them.

Remember that while all psychotropic medications can cause *sedation* (the side effect of sleepiness or grogginess), usually it is related to the *amount* of the particular medication taken. If the amount of medication is lowered a little bit, the sedation typically disappears. Parents often tell me, "I don't want my child to be a zombie." I respond that I don't want their child to be a zombie either. Part of my job, and every psychiatrist's job, is searching to find a dosage of the proper medication that will produce its benefits with no sedation.

In the past couple of years some of the most frequently used medications in children and adolescents have received the US Food and Drug Administration (FDA) Black Box warning. This list has included the selective serotonin reuptake inhibitors (SSRIs) and other antidepressants used to treat depression and anxiety disorders (see medication groups 2 and 4 below), as well as all the stimulant medications, and some non-stimulant medications, used to treat attention deficit hyperactivity disorder (ADHD) (see medication group 1 below).

The Black Box type of warning (over 325 medications have them) is found on the printed insert accompanying medications and gets its name because the warning is enclosed in a rectangular black box, to draw attention to it. While there are usually long lists of cautions and warnings given on most medications, the Black Box warning is the strongest type given by the FDA. The number of scientific studies on medication use in children and adolescents are fewer than in adults and very few in number relative to how widely the medications are used. The Black Box warning often includes information indicating the noteworthy risks of using the medication in a child or adolescent. It may indicate that there are not sufficient studies supporting the medication's use in children and adolescents and consequently no approval is given for its use in the pediatric population. The antidepressants and stimulants have been, and still are, widely used, but the Black Box warnings have resulted in an increase in the caution with which they are used. Medication used in a way that is not fully approved by the FDA is considered *off label* (see discussion under antidepressants on page 224 for more perspective on this). It is important for you to be clear about what the side effect warnings mean and what the most important side effects to be alert to are. Ask about and discuss these with your child's doctor.

Once your child has started on medication, *your physician, you, and your child should work together to assess the balance of the desired beneficial effects and the undesired side effects*. This is easy when the benefits may be clear and the side effects either not present or minimal. It is also easy, although disappointing, when the benefits are not present and the negative side effects prominent. It is harder to decide when either of the following is true:

- both benefits and side effects are equally present
- initially the benefits seem to outweigh the unwanted side effects but, some time during treatment, the balance shifts.

During those times I usually recommend waiting a bit of time to see if the side effect will decrease. If the side effect is too distressing, waiting may not be an option. Then another medication with a different side effect profile would be tried. In the near future, an inexpensive blood test will be available to help a doctor decide whether or not a particular individual is more or less susceptible to side effects from a particular medication.

Medications, and the side effects of medications for mental health problems

The following material, based upon my clinical experience and knowledge of the professional literature, provides information to help you and your child understand more about conventional medications. For each of the five categories of symptoms, I list the medications used to treat those symptoms and their side effects (common and serious).

I do not list the side effects for each specific brand of medication. Rather, I focus on the group of medications that share a common treatment focus. (This is not true of the mood stabilizers group, since in that group, each medication has a somewhat distinctive side effect profile.) For information on a specific brand of medicine, look at the insert that comes with the particular medication your child is taking, or ask your doctor or pharmacist.

Below I list the medication groups and the corresponding five main categories of symptoms for which they are used:

1. medication for symptoms of inattention, impulsivity, hyperactivity, and distractibility (Tables 9.1 and 9.2)

2. medication for symptoms of depression (Table 9.3)

3. medication for symptoms of bipolar disorder and severe mood instability (Table 9.4)

4. medications for symptoms of anxiety (Table 9.5)

5. medications for symptoms of psychosis (schizophrenia, paranoia), severe mood disorder (severe depression or mood instability/bipolar disorder), severe anxiety, severe aggression, severe agitation, and Tourette's syndrome (Table 9.6).

In my explanations below, I generally put the most commonly used name of the medication first. Sometimes that first name of the medication is a brand name; other times it is generic. I put the *generic name* in *italics* and the *brand name* takes an *initial capital*. Text that follows each table expands upon the information presented.

1. Inattention, impulsivity, hyperactivity, and distractibility

This medication group includes a number of the well-known stimulant medications, used for the treatment of ADHD, with and without hyperactivity. The main difference between these medicines is the length of time that each medication is effective and whether it is similar to Ritalin (*methylphenidate*) or to Dexedrine (*amphetamine*).

The benefits from stimulants can be seen quickly, often within hours, when the proper dosage is reached. The patch takes about 1.5 hours to work and lasts about three hours after taking it off, thus the coverage is quite flexible. Stimulants generally are well tolerated. They are more likely to have benefits than serious side effects, and usually any side effects are seen quickly.

However, it is important to inform your child's primary-care doctor if there is a history of cardiovascular disease or sudden death of unknown cause in a family member before the age of 40, or if your child has a heart structural abnormality (hole in the heart) or any symptoms of chest pain, dizziness or lightheadedness associated with exercise. With this information, your child's doctor will be in a better position to determine if stimulants are the right drug to use.

Some children taking these medications may develop *tics*: involuntary small motor movements of the face, neck, or upper body. The tics tend to stop when the medication is stopped. If significant tics do develop, you, your child, and the doctor may decide to continue the stimulant and add another medicine to help decrease the tics.

Table 9.1 Stimulant medication for inattention, impulsivity, and hyperactivity and their side effects

Types of stimulant medication	Ritalin-type (methylphenidate)	Amphetamine-type (dextroamphetamine)
Specific medications of short duration	Ritalin-type stimulants lasting 3–5 hours: Generic Ritalin/ *methylphenidate* Focalin	Amphetamine-type stimulant lasting 4–6 hours: Generic Dexedrine/ *dextroamphetamine*
Specific medications of intermediate duration	Ritalin-type stimulants lasting 6–8 hours: Metadate ER (5–6 hours) Ritalin ER Metadate CD (6–8 hours)	Amphetamine-type stimulant lasting 4–6 hours: Adderall
Specific medications of extended duration	Ritalin-type stimulants lasting up to 12 hours: Concerta (10–12 hours) Ritalin LA (8–12 hours) Focalin XR (8–12 hours) Daytrana, a patch, (variable: 2–12 hours)	Amphetamine-type stimulant lasting up to 12 hours: Adderall XR (10–12 hours) Vyvanse (*lisdexamfetamine*) (12 hours)

Partial list of *common* side effects that can occur in all stimulants. For most symptoms listed, occurrence is in less than one in ten patients. *Severity varies* from mild to great: decreased appetite, tics, stomach and headaches, anxiety, trouble sleeping.

Partial list of *serious* side effects that can occur in all stimulants. For most symptoms listed, occurrence is in less than one in 100 patients, often in less than one in 1000: Abnormal heart rhythm, seizure, stroke, heart attack, psychosis, Tourette's syndrome.

Or you might all decide to stop the stimulant medication and try some other medicine that may not be quite as effective but does not cause tics.

Your child does not have to have regular blood testing while on these medications (unless he is on other medications that require tests). Some experts are concerned that long-term usage of these stimulants may affect children's growth. Others are not as concerned, citing that no net long-term negative effect on growth has been convincingly shown.

While the stimulants can be abused, there is no indication that taking these medications properly causes drug abuse. In fact, studies have shown a decreased likelihood of substance abuse for those with ADHD who are treated, in contrast to those not treated. Vyvanse is a new form of amphetamine less likely to be abused because of the way it is metabolized in the body.

Table 9.2 Non-stimulant medication for inattention, impulsivity, and hyperactivity and their side effects

Types of non-stimulant medication	Noradrenergic reuptake inhibitor non-stimulant	Alpha agonist type non-stimulant	Antidepressant type non-stimulant
Specific medications and duration of action	Strattera (atomoxetine) lasts 24 hours	Clonidine, lasts 4 hours Tenex (guanfacine) lasts 6–12 hours	Wellbutrin (buproprion) lasts 24 hours
Partial list of common side effects. For most symptoms listed, occurrence is in less than one in ten patients. **Severity varies** from mild to great.	Dry mouth, stomach aches, trouble sleeping, constipation, fatigue, dizziness	Dry mouth, dizziness, tiredness, constipation, low blood pressure	Nausea, trouble sleeping, dry mouth, tremor, headache, agitation, blurry vision
Partial list of serious side effects. For most symptoms listed, occurrence is in less than one in 100 patients and often in less than one in 1000.	Increased blood pressure, liver toxicity, suicidal thoughts	Severe rebound hypertension if stopped abruptly	Seizures, abnormal heart rhythm, suicidality, psychosis, severe skin reactions

Below I provide more detail about each non-stimulant.

Strattera (*atomoxetine*), a *noradrenergic* reuptake inhibitor type medication, is a non-stimulant used to treat attentional and hyperactivity disorder symptoms. It has some noteworthy advantages and differences with the stimulants.

- It lasts 24 hours and needs to be taken only one or two times each day. Thus it can be particularly helpful to a child with trouble focusing on tasks to be done in the morning.

- It is less likely to cause anxiety than the stimulants. Thus it may be preferred when attention problems are accompanied by moodiness and anxiety.

- It does not seem to cause tics and therefore may be helpful for a child with Tourette's syndrome.

- It may be used alone for milder symptoms or along with the stimulant type medications for more intense symptoms.

- It does not require blood tests. Negative effects on appetite and sleep seem to be less frequent than with the stimulant medication.

- It does not seem to be as effective as stimulants to help with more severe impulsivity or hyperactivity.

Clonidine (Catapres) and Tenex (*guanfacine*), both in the category of alpha agonists, have the advantage over stimulants of not causing an increase in anxiety. These medications:

- may be used alone or added to stimulants if a high level of hyperactivity, anxiety, and aggressiveness is present
- are generally well tolerated, and may have an effect within days or a week, assuming a proper dosage has been attained
- may cause excessive sedation, which is addressed by decreasing the dosage
- should be started and stopped slowly—they can have the unwanted side effect of lowering blood pressure if the dose is increased too quickly or raising blood pressure if the dose is lowered too abruptly
- should best be started after an electrocardiogram (ECG) is obtained. This is to make sure a child has no heart-rhythm abnormality that might be worsened by the medication.

Wellbutrin (*bupropion*) is an antidepressant non-stimulant. It:

- may be used when stimulants are not effective or when depression is prominent and ADHD less prominent
- is generally well tolerated
- should be used in high doses cautiously. There is concern about a *seizure* occurring, especially if other factors are present in the patient that might lead to a seizure (such as epilepsy, anorexia, or bulimia).

2. Depression

Medications for mood are divided into two groups. The first group (Table 9.3) comprises *antidepressants*, which are medications used to treat the symptoms of depression (such as low mood, low energy, disrupted sleep, and suicidal thoughts). The second group (Table 9.4) comprises *mood stabilizers*. These are used to treat the symptoms of bipolar disorder or severe mood instability (such as erratic, elevated, or highly irritable moods that alternate with, or mix with, depression). Once a therapeutic dosage has been reached, the speed of onset of most antidepressant medication varies from ten days to a few weeks.

Selective serotonin reuptake inhibitors (SSRIs):

- are the most commonly used first-choice antidepressants for children and adolescents because they are better tolerated and safer in overdosage than other antidepressants
- have a high benefit to side effect profile, meaning that the benefits outweigh the side effects.

In 2004, some research and practice doctors raised concerns about the frequency of the serious side effects of suicidal thoughts and behavior in children taking the SSRI

Table 9.3 Medications for symptoms of depression and their side effects

Types of antidepressant medication	SSRI and SSRI like antidepressants	Dual action antidepressants	Uncategorized antidepressant	Tricyclic antidepressants
Specific types of antidepressants	Prozac (*fluoxetine*) Zoloft (*sertraline*) Paxil (*paroxitine*) Celexa (*citalopram*) Lexapro (*escitalopram*) Remeron (*mirtazapine*)	Effexor (*venlafaxine*) Cymbalta (*duloxetine*)	Wellbutrin (*bupropion*)	Tofranil (*imipramine*) Pamelor (*nortriptyline*) Norpramin (*desipramine*)
Partial list of* common *side effects for the different groups of antidepressants. Most symptoms listed occur in less than one in ten patients, but some occur in one in five patients. ***Severity varies*** from mild to great.	Nausea, headache, sleep problems, anxiety, tiredness, loss of appetite, tremor, sweating, decreased libido, other sexual problems	Nausea, headache, dizziness, sleep problems, constipation, anxiety, tiredness, impotence, hypertension	Nausea, trouble sleeping, dry mouth, tremor, headache, agitation, blurry vision	Drowsiness, dry mouth, dizziness, constipation, blurred vision, palpitations, increased appetite, nausea, urinary problems
Partial list of* serious *side effects for the different groups of antidepressants. They are infrequent; most symptoms listed occur in less than one in 100 patients and some occur in one in 1000 patients.	Worsening of depression, suicidality, seizures, mania, severe rash, withdrawal symptoms, abnormal motor movements	Worsening of depression, suicidality, seizures, psychosis, severe hypertension, withdrawal symptoms, abnormal motor movements	Worsening of depression, suicidality, seizures, abnormal heart rhythm, suicidality, psychosis, mania, severe skin reactions	Worsening of depression, suicidality, abnormal heart rhythm, heart attack, stroke, seizure, psychosis, mania, paralyzed small colon

Paxil. British researchers reported that children who had been on Paxil had more suicidal thoughts and behavior than expected. They recommended that Paxil no longer be used with children and adolescents. But if a child had been on Paxil for a long time and it had been helpful, it was thought reasonable for the doctor and parent to decide to keep a child on the medication.

After the concern about Paxil, a similar worry was raised about all the SSRIs (except Prozac). This concern was promoted by reports of increased suicidal ideation and behavior in some children after taking these other medications. This increase seems closely related to the response of an increase in feelings of agitation and tension that some individuals have when first going on these medications. This may show up as feeling the need to keep moving, for example, pacing or tapping, and has been described as, "feeling like I want to jump out of my skin."

With this new understanding of the prevalence of such worrisome side effects, experts debated how much caution was needed in the use of these medications in children and adolescents. Some individuals wanted to stop the prescription of these medications completely for children and adolescents. Because these medications can be extremely helpful, others thought they should not be removed from use.

Most clinicians, myself included, believe that:

- with careful usage, the overall benefits of these medications far outweigh the small likelihood of making things worse
- close monitoring for a worsening of symptoms, such as increased suicidal ideation and agitation especially during the first three months, is strongly recommended
- since milder side effects often disappear, a doctor may reasonably recommend sticking with the SSRI antidepressant for a few weeks to see if beneficial effects will occur or increase and the worrisome side effects decrease or disappear
- further scientific investigation of this matter continues.

Routine blood tests are usually not performed with SSRIs, nor is an ECG required. Below I describe other specific medications used to treat symptoms of depression.

Effexor (*venlafaxine*):
- can be helpful even if the SSRIs haven't been
- has a faster onset of positive benefits than that of most other antidepressants
- may cause an elevation of *blood pressure*, which is monitored by checking your child's blood pressure during the first week or so of starting Effexor and then again when there is a dosage increase
- does not require regular blood testing or an ECG.

Wellbutrin (*bupropion*):
- can be quite helpful even if the SSRIs haven't been

- may, in high doses, cause *seizures*; this concern is increased if other factors are also present in the patient that might lead to a seizure (such as epilepsy or an eating disorder)
- does not require regular blood testing or an ECG.

Tricyclic antidepressants:

- provide positive results and few side effects for some children and more mixed or negative ones for others
- sometimes cause dry mouth, constipation, and lightheadedness on arising quickly, although lowering the dose may result in fewer of these side effects
- are usually started after an ECG. A child who might have even a slight heart abnormality does not take these medications
- are used less frequently than SSRIs because of the possible cardiac and other side effects.

If a child psychiatrist seriously thinks that your depressed child might have a bipolar mood disorder:

- he may not use antidepressants for the depressive side of a bipolar mood disorder but rather rely on a mood stabilizer to address the depression
- he may not use an antidepressant alone because the erratic and irritable mood states of a child with bipolar disorder may worsen
- he may want to use an antidepressant along with a mood stabilizer.

3. Bipolar disorder and severe mood instability

The *mood stabilizing medications* listed in Table 9.4 include lithium, the anti-epileptic drugs (AED) and the antipsychotic medications. These medications may also be used for extreme irritability and aggressiveness, even without other clear indications of a mood instability disorder.

The designation of "first line/choice" for the anti-epileptic drugs generally means:

- the medication has been used extensively
- its effectiveness has been proven through rigorous scientific studies.

The designation of "second line/choice" means:

- the medication is relatively new in use as a mood stabilizer
- its effectiveness, when used alone, has not been sufficiently substantiated through scientific studies.

Lithium:

- comes in short (*lithium carbonate*) and long-acting (Eskalith, Lithobid) forms

Table 9.4 Medications for symptoms of bipolar disorder/severe mood instability and their side effects

Types of mood stabilizers	Lithium	Anti-epileptic Drugs of first choice	Anti-epileptic Drugs of second choice	Atypical Anti-psychotics
Specific mood stabilizers	Eskalith Lithobid (*lithium carbonate*)	Tegretol (*carbamazepine*) Depakote (*divalproex*) Depakene (*valproic acid*) Lamictal (*lamotrigine*)	Gabitril (*tiagabine*) Neurontin (*gabapentin*) Topomax (*topiramate*) Trileptal (*oxcarbazapine*)	Abilify Geodon Risperdal Seroquel Zyprexa Clozaril
Partial list of **common** *side effects* for the different groups of mood stabilizers. Most symptoms listed occur in less than one in ten patients, but some occur in one in five patients. *Severity varies* from mild to great.	Tremor, frequent urination, diarrhea, nausea, drowsiness, muscle weakness, blurred vision, weight gain, worsening acne	Headache, nausea, weight gain, tiredness, diarrhea, hair loss, visual abnormalities, elevation of liver enzymes, dizziness	Tiredness, dizziness, walking shakily, tiredness, blurred vision, nausea	See Table 9.6
Partial list of **serious** *side effects* for the different groups of mood stabilizers. They are infrequent; most symptoms listed occur in less than one in 100 patients and some occur in one in 1000 patients.	Seizures, abnormal heart rhythm, thyroid disorder, kidney dysfunction, increased white cells, increased pressure inside the skull	Inflammation of the liver or pancreas, severe suppression of red or white cells, severe toxic skin reactions, congenital abnormalities	Low white cell count (Neurontin), seizures (Gabitril), abnormalities of bone and blood chemistries, skin and liver toxicity (Topomax), similar to Tegretol, but less frequent (Trileptal)	See Table 9.6

- is a naturally occurring element, and thus is distinct from the other man-made mood-stabilizing medications
- was the first medication to have a significant impact on bipolar disorder, with widespread usage beginning before the 1970s, yet it continues to be a first-line choice for treating mood instability
- has a side effect profile that is different from other mood stabilizers

- has a proper dose that is determined by noting how much improvement there has been at a particular dose and by measuring the blood level of lithium

- has a narrow range between the amount in the blood that is helpful and the amount that causes toxic side effects

- requires your child's doctor to keep a close eye on your child's lithium blood level, because the blood level can change, even once a proper dosage has been attained

- can build up into a toxic range (that can be measured in the blood) because of certain medications, and some physical states (like dehydration due to excessive sweating or diarrhea)

- has toxic effects from too much of it being in the body that include:

  - excessive thirst and urination

  - tremor

  - altered states of consciousness.

Long-term usage of lithium can affect the thyroid and kidney:

- Your child's treating physician will monitor lithium's effect on the thyroid and kidney through various periodic blood tests.

- The disruption of thyroid function may be treated with a small dose of thyroid medication. This may or may not need to continue if lithium is discontinued. Experts disagree about whether lithium causes an abnormality of the thyroid or simply triggers an underlying problem.

- Similar uncertainty is present about lithium's effect upon the kidney. If your doctor notes some negative effect on your child's kidney over the long term, he will generally discontinue the lithium when the problem is discovered.

AEDs as mood stabilizers:

- were first used as a remedy for seizures and therefore are referred to as "anti-epileptic drugs" and "mood stabilizing drugs"

- like lithium, can produce seemingly miraculous changes

- all have the potential for serious or even (rare) life-threatening side effects

- under proper monitoring, are reasonably safe, cause serious side effects in a very small percentage of patients, and often offer the only available relief.

Next I describe specific AED mood-stabilizing medications.

Depakote (*divalproex*):

- may be substituted for by a similar chemical form called Depakene (*valproic acid*)
- has a proper dose that is determined by noting how much improvement there has been at a particular dose and by measuring the blood level of Depakote through periodic blood tests
- is monitored through periodic blood tests to avoid toxic levels and to check for possible side effects on the liver
- has weight gain as a common side effect.

Some serious side effects for Depakote cannot be monitored through blood tests. Thus your child's doctors rely on you to bring attention to certain physical complaints such as:

- acute abdominal pain (possible pancreatitis)
- significant changes in menstrual cycle (possible dysfunctional ovaries).

Tegretol (*carbamazepine*):

- is monitored through periodic blood tests to avoid toxic levels and to check for possible side effects on the liver and blood system.

Some serious side effects for Tegretol cannot be adequately monitored through blood tests. Thus your child's doctors rely on you to bring attention to certain physical complaints such as:

- a bad sore throat and high fever (possibly due to a low white cell count)
- a rash, especially early in treatment (possible start of severe skin reaction).

Lamictal (*lamotrigine*):

- has a proper dose that is determined only by noting how much improvement there has been at a particular dose and *not* by measuring the blood level through periodic blood tests
- must be raised in dosage *very slowly*. Doing so quickly increases the possibility of developing a rare and serious potentially life-threatening rash
- may produce a rash that is particularly worrisome if accompanied by a fever, sore throat, or neck and facial involvement with puffy eyes.

Trileptal (*oxcarbazine*):

- is closely related to Tegretol, but less often has serious side effects
- does not require monitoring for blood level
- has the main concerning side effect of excessive sedation
- is often chosen because it has few serious side effects, even though it has not been as consistently effective as Tegretol for stabilizing mood.

Neurontin (*gabapentin*), Topomax (*topiramate*), and Gabitril (*tiagabine*):

- Neurontin (*gabapentin*) and Topomax (*topiramate*) do not require blood monitoring.

- Neurontin (*gabapentin*) has few serious side effects, although raising the dose rapidly may cause excessive sedation.

- Topomax (*topiramate*) can cause weight loss. Therefore, it may be used along with a mood stabilizer that can cause weight gain.

- Topomax (*topiramate*) may cause excessive sedation and memory difficulties, as well as bone and blood chemistry abnormalities.

- Gabitril (*tiagabine*) is a recent addition to this group of anti-epileptics, and its level of effectiveness in treating mood instability has not been clearly defined.

Atypical antipsychotics:

- are used increasingly for the treatment of mood disorders that are either intense or extreme, or are not responding well enough to the AED and lithium mood stabilizers or antidepressants alone

- are medications that are contrasted with the "typical" (or "conventional") antipsychotics (see Table 9.6), which are generally not used as mood stabilizers

- also are referred to as *major tranquilizers*, since they are used in so many different circumstances—mood disorders of the depressive or bipolar type, severe anxiety, severe agitation or aggression, and Tourette's syndrome.

4. Anxiety

The medications below are used to address the feelings of intense anxiety and fear. These feelings may come up in many different circumstances and settings and may be accompanied by a range of different thoughts and behaviors.

These medications may be appropriate if your child's worries:

- are present for much of your child's waking life. He may be diagnosed as having a *generalized anxiety disorder*

- suddenly become intensely frightening, and your child feels overwhelmed and has to flee. He may be suffering from *panic attacks*. If such episodes occur repeatedly, he may be diagnosed as having a *panic disorder*

- occur primarily when your child is separated from you (like when he goes to school or has a sleep-over at a friend's house). He might be suffering from *separation anxiety*

- appear as intense shyness that leads to his avoiding contact with peers or adults whenever possible. He may have a *social phobia*

- show up as his being very preoccupied with particular, often frightening, ideas or topics (obsessions), which occur along with the need to do repetitive behaviors (compulsions), that are used to counteract those frightening ideas. He may be diagnosed as having an *obsessive –compulsive disorder.*

Table 9.5A Antidepressant medications for symptoms of anxiety and their side effects

Type of antidepressant for anxiety and type of anxiety treated	SSRIs (for all types of anxiety)	Tricyclic antidepressants (for separation anxiety or obsessions and compulsions)	Other antidepressants (for generalized anxiety)
Specific medications	Prozac (*fluoxetine*) Zoloft (*sertraline*) Paxil (*paroxitine*) Celexa (*citalopram*) Lexapro (*escitalopram*) Remeron (*mirtazapine*)	Tofranil (*imipramine*) Norpramin (*desipramine*) + others (for separation anxiety) Anafranil (*clomipramine*) (for obsessions and compulsions)	Effexor (*venlafaxine*)
Partial list of common side effects. Most symptoms listed occur in less than one in ten patients, but some occur in one in five patients. **Severity varies** from mild to great.	Nausea, headache, sleep problems, anxiety, tiredness, loss of appetite, tremor, sweating, decreased libido, other sexual problems	See Table 9.3	See Table 9.3
Partial list of serious side effects. They are infrequent; most symptoms listed occur in less than one in 100 patients and some occur in one in 1000 patients.	Onset or worsening of depression, suicidality, seizures, mania, severe rash, withdrawal symptoms, abnormal motor movements	Onset or worsening of depression, suicidality, abnormal heart rhythm, heart attack, stroke, seizure, psychosis, mania, paralyzed small colon	Onset or worsening of depression, suicidality, abnormal heart rhythm, heart attack, stroke, seizure, psychosis, mania, paralyzed small colon

All of these situations are linked by unusually intense and disruptive anxiety, which may benefit from the use of medication. It is noteworthy that:

- many of the previously noted antidepressants, such as the SSRIs, are used to treat this range of symptoms (less for generalized anxiety)

- generalized anxiety may be more effectively treated with the antidepressant, Effexor.

Table 9.5B Other medications for symptoms of anxiety and their side effects

Type of anti-anxiety medication and symptoms treated	Benzodiazepines (for panic and specific anxiety provoking situations)	Non-benzodiazepine (for generalized anxiety)
Specific medications	Ativan (*lorazepam*) Klonopin (*clonazepam*) Valium (*diazepam*) Xanax (*alprazolam*) + others	BuSpar (*buspirone*)
Partial list of **common** *side effects* for the different groups of anti-anxiety medications. Most symptoms listed occur in less than one in ten patients, but some occur in one in five patients. *Severity varies* from mild to great.	Drowsiness, confusion, walk unsteadily, headache, memory problems, low blood pressure depression, sleep changes	Dizziness, drowsiness, headache, nausea, dry mouth, decreased concentration
Partial list of **serious** *side effects* for the different groups of anti-anxiety medications. They are infrequent; most symptoms listed occur in less than one in 100 patients and some occur in one in 1000 patients.	Depressed breathing, low white cell count, liver toxicity, dependency/abuse	May occur but none reported

Below I describe specific medications in this category.

SSRIs:

- are the most commonly used first choice medication for children and adolescents with symptoms of panic attacks, social phobias, and obsessions/compulsions
- are better tolerated and thought to be safer in overdosage than many other antidepressants
- usually require a higher dosage to treat anxiety symptoms than for symptoms of depression alone
- have a speed of beginning the improvement of symptoms that varies from ten days to a few weeks, once a therapeutic dosage has been reached

- generally have a high benefit to side effect profile (meaning that the benefits outweigh the side effects)
- may cause headache, gastrointestinal upset, and some initial jitteriness or agitation.

Because of the new understanding of the prevalence of the worrisome side effects of increased suicidal ideation and behavior in some children after taking SSRIs, experts have recommended caution any time these medications are used. (See more detailed discussion of SSRIs in the section on antidepressants—for background history.) Any increase in feelings of agitation and tension, which some individuals may have when first going on these medications, should be closely monitored. This agitation may show up as feeling the need to keep moving, for example, pacing or tapping, and has been described as, "feeling like I want to jump out of my skin." It may be confused with a worsening of the anxiety symptom. Because these medications can be extremely helpful, and the incidence of this problem seems low, the medications are still widely in use.

Most clinicians, myself included, believe that:

- with careful usage, the overall benefits of these medications far outweigh the small likelihood of making things worse
- *children on such medications must be closely monitored* for a worsening of symptoms, such as the appearance of suicidal ideation or increased agitation, especially during the first three months
- since some milder degree side effects often disappear, a doctor may reasonably recommend sticking with the SSRI for a few weeks to see if beneficial effects will occur or increase and side effects decrease
- in some children with a tendency towards mood instability, an SSRI used to treat anxiety may cause increased agitation and an erratic or labile mood. This kind of response may lead to the use of a mood stabilizer or other anti-anxiety medications.

Routine blood tests are usually not performed with SSRIs, nor is an ECG required.

Tricyclic antidepressants:

- work well and with few side effects for some children with separation anxiety; other children have a more mixed or negative experience
- may be used to treat anxiety in children with ADHD
- sometimes cause dry mouth, constipation, and lightheadedness on arising quickly. Lowering the dose may result in fewer side effects
- are started *after* an ECG. A child who might have some heart abnormality does not take these medications

- are used less frequently than SSRIs because of possible cardiac and other side effects
- include only one tricyclic, *clomipramine* (Anafranil), that is used to treat obsessive–compulsive disorder
- when used to treat anxiety in some children with a tendency towards mood instability, they may cause increased agitation and an erratic or labile mood. This response may lead to the use of a mood stabilizer or other anti-anxiety medications.

Effexor (*venlafaxine*):
- can be helpful for generalized anxiety
- has the main worrisome side effect at higher doses of an elevation of blood pressure, which is monitored by testing your child's blood pressure during the first week or so of starting Effexor and then again when there is a dosage increase
- does not require regular blood testing or a preliminary ECG.

Benzodiazepines:
- are used very cautiously in young children (under eight or nine) since these medications can sometimes cause a young child to become more agitated
- are also used cautiously in adolescents, since these medications are habit forming and can be abused
- may cause excessive sedation when given in high doses—this can be decreased by adjusting the dosage
- have a high benefit to low side effect ratio (meaning that the benefits outweigh the side effects)
- should *never* be taken with alcohol.

Non-benzodiazepine, BuSpar (*buspirone*):
- is chemically different from the benzodiazepines, and somewhat similar to the SSRIs
- may take a few weeks at a particular dose to produce positive effects
- is limited mostly to use in generalized anxiety—it is not helpful for panic or sudden anxiety (in contrast to the benzodiazepines)
- is often used along with an SSRI or other medication
- may cause gastrointestinal (stomach) upset
- does not cause increased agitation in younger children, nor is it habit forming or a drug of abuse
- requires neither blood tests nor ECG for routine use.

5. Psychosis, severe mood disorder, severe anxiety, severe aggression, severe agitation, and Tourette's syndrome

Psychotic symptoms—such as hallucinations, paranoid thinking, or delusions (see Chapter 2)—may be treated with the older antipsychotics, but would more likely be treated with newer antipsychotics, also called the "atypical antipsychotics." The newer medications have a wider range of positive effects and fewer neurological side effects. Some of the newer medications may also be used for extremes of mood, anxiety, aggressiveness, and hyperactivity.

Table 9.6 Medication for symptoms of psychosis/ other extreme symptoms and their side effects

Type of antipsychotic	Older, "typical"	Newer, "atypical"
Specific medications	Haldol (*haloperidol*) Mellaril (*thioridazine*) Thorazine (*chlorpromazine*) Trilafon (*perphenazine*) Stelazine (*trifluoperazine*) + many others	Abilify (*aripiprazole*) Clozaril (*clozapine*) Geodon (*ziprasidone*) Risperdal (*risperidone*) Seroquel (*quetiapine*) Zyprexa (*olanzapine*)
Partial list of common side effects for the different groups of anti-psychotic medications. Most occur in less than one in ten patients, but some occur in one in five patients. **Severity varies**: mild to great.	Short-term abnormal movements and restlessness; sleepiness, dry mouth, constipation, breast tenderness and discharge; menstrual abnormalities; sun burn easily	Headache, dizziness, tiredness, weight gain, dry mouth, constipation, menstrual abnormalities, increased cholesterol
Partial list of serious side effects for the different groups of anti-psychotic medications. They are infrequent; most listed occur in less than one in 100 patients and some occur in one in 1000 patients.	Long-lasting or permanent abnormal muscle tics and movements, acute toxic reaction, seizures, heat stroke	Diabetes, stroke, heart disease

Below, I refer to these medications (both the typical and atypical) as *major tranquilizers*, not only as "antipsychotic medications." This is because even though these medications were first developed to treat psychosis (schizophrenia, paranoia, psychotic depression and mania), they are now often used in a wide range of disorders and situations for which the term psychosis is misleading.

The older types of antipsychotics/major tranquilizers:

- are still in use when there is no response to the newer major tranquilizers or when there is some specific indication for using them
- are less expensive than the newer major tranquilizers

- may produce neurological side effects that show up as muscular tics or spasms. These movements may occur 1. shortly after starting the medicine and usually disappear with the help of another medicine or on their own, or may occur 2. after long-term treatment (and are called tardive dyskinesia), but these may then not be reversible
- may cause an increase in a hormone that enlarges breast size and causes breast fluid discharge or disrupts the menstrual cycle
- raise less concern than the newer atypical medications about the long-term effects upon the cardiovascular system, blood sugar regulating system, and the body's management of cholesterol and lipids.

The newer atypical antipsychotics/major tranquilizers:

- have been used extensively over the last ten years
- do not require close blood monitoring, except for Clozaril (clozapine), which can cause very serious negative effects on the blood cell system (particularly the white cells)
- have a low incidence of neurological side effects and seem to be well tolerated
- recently have been associated with concerns about how long-term usage influences the body's metabolism
- can negatively affect the cardiovascular system, the blood sugar regulating system, and the body's management of cholesterol and lipids
- can cause a lot of weight gain and associated negative metabolic effects (Risperdal, Zyprexa, Seroquel, and Clozaril). This is less the case with Geodon and Abilify.

Table 9.7 (below) provides a quick outline of the primary and secondary areas of treatment for some of the most commonly used medications in child pharmacotherapy: the antidepressants, the mood stabilizers, the atypical antipsychotics, and the stimulants.

6. Medications for other specific disorders or symptoms

Tic disorder:

- usually refers to the disorder of Tourette's syndrome
- may be treated with medications as varied as Clonidine, Tenex (*guanfacine*), Haldol, Risperdal, benzodiazepines, or some SSRIs.

Sleep disorders:

- most commonly involve ongoing difficulty falling asleep
- may be helped by the same medication treating the primary problem, such as an antidepressant or antipsychotic

Table 9.7 Summary overview of medication and common areas of use

Medication	Inattention, impulsivity, hyperactivity and distractibility	Depression	Bipolar disorder and severe mood instability	Anxiety	Psychosis and severe symptoms of mood, anxiety, aggression, and agitation
SSRIs		P		P	
Effexor		P		P	
Wellbutrin	S	P			
Tricyclics	S	P		S	
AED and lithium mood stabilizers		S	P		
Atypical antipsychotics		S	P		P
Stimulants	P				

P = primary usage in this area; S = secondary use in this area

- may be helped by medication with sedation as a side effect, such as Benadryl (*diphenhydramine*), Vistaril/Atarax (*hydoxyzine*), *clonidine* (Catapres), Tofranil (*imipramine*), or Desyrel (*trazodone*).

Bedwetting:

- may be remedied with the use of Tofranil, DDAVP, or Ditropan
- can also be helped by a training device that wakes your child at the first indication of bedwetting. The device consists of a moisture-detecting sensor, one end of which is attached to your child's pajamas and the other end is attached to a buzzer that goes off as soon as a drop of urine touches the sensor. The device helps your child become aware of being wet, and this, along with encouragement, ultimately leads to waking at the first sign of needing to urinate.

Eating disorders:

- may be treated by the use of SSRIs
- may also be helped by other medications that address any accompanying symptoms, such as depression, panic, or obsessive thoughts.

Post-traumatic stress disorder:

- may be treated with SSRIs, mood stabilizers, and atypical antipsychotics
- may be treated by medication to address a specific symptom—such as terror, depression, mood swings, flashbacks, and intrusive images, or insomnia—that is part of the disorder.

Pharmacotherapy: frequently asked questions

The following questions and responses may help you make more informed decisions regarding pharmacotherapy.

1. Who is the best person to provide medication treatment for my child, and why?

The best person is an experienced clinician who meets the following criteria:

- is able to do a sophisticated clinical evaluation of your child from a psychological and medical perspective
- has expert knowledge and lots of experience with the use of medications that address disturbed emotions and behavior in children.

Child psychiatrists meet these criteria best. But because of the shortage of child psychiatrists, this specialist may not be immediately available. A pediatrician, family practitioner, developmental pediatrician, or adult psychiatrist also can provide pharmacotherapy for your child. Over the past few years, some nurses, called clinical nurse specialists, have had training in psychiatric pharmacotherapy and practice under the supervision of a psychiatrist. Such a nurse may provide the medication treatment needed for your child, particularly if you are being seen in a clinic.

If the best trained specialist is not available, but the situation is complicated, you could choose to have your child begin treatment with another specialist and then transfer to a child psychiatrist when an opening is available. Your child's pediatrician, family practitioner, or adult psychiatrist may get ongoing consultation with your child's therapist and a child psychiatrist colleague regarding the best treatment. These alternatives are not the preferred routes, but may be all that is available at the time your child needs medication.

2. How do I decide to have my child take medication? Does my child take medication with, or instead of, psychotherapy?

If your child's symptoms are in the more serious range and your child is in a lot of ongoing distress, then it is appropriate to consider medication in addition to psychotherapy. Medication is warranted if:

- your child's life is so disrupted that she cannot attend school
- she cannot engage with peers

- there is an ongoing threat to your child's own safety or that of others
- she functions okay but is in great emotional distress.

When symptoms are mild or moderate, I tend to "wait and see" if psychotherapy is helpful enough on its own. When symptoms are severe, distress is high, and intense worry is evident, I am more likely to recommend medication at, or shortly after, the start of therapy.

The question of using medication *instead* of psychotherapy goes in the wrong direction. If your child is having symptoms severe enough to consider medication, your child should also have some form of psychotherapy. If you put your child on medication without trying psychotherapy, you are vastly shortchanging your child and your family. Medication ought to be "in addition to" rather than "instead of" psychotherapy. Medication and psychotherapy offer different approaches to problems and are helpful in different ways. They are complementary, not interchangeable.

3. How do I tell whether the medication is helping?

Look for a decrease in intensity, duration, and frequency of the problematic behavior or emotional state. Sometimes changes are quite dramatic, but most often they are gradual and progressive.

Unlike many antibiotics or other types of medications for bodily ills, one dose does not "fit all" with psychotropic medications. Some medications, such as the stimulants, may produce a change in your child's behavior within days of getting a proper dose. But finding that proper dose may take a couple of weeks or more. Some medications, such as the antidepressants, may take up to a few weeks to show positive changes, even when at a proper dose. Other medications may take even longer. That's why there may be frequent brief appointments to evaluate the effectiveness of the medication and make changes, particularly during the beginning of pharmacotherapy.

Chart specific behaviors you are hoping to see change with the help of medication. Report these changes to your child's doctor during the visit. Sometimes a doctor will decide that the maximum reasonable dose has been tried and that it is time to try another medication. With most mood stabilizers, the doctor may assess the symptoms and measure the level of the medicine in your child's blood as a guide for the optimal dose.

If your doctor has tried different medications with no success, you may feel discouraged. But don't simply let the matter drop. Share your disappointment and discouragement with your doctor; tell him your doubts and your uncertainties. The doctor needs your feedback to do the best job possible, particularly when things don't seem to be going well.

4. How long will pharmacotherapy last?

Once improvement has happened and your child seems "his old self" or better, he will commonly stay on the medication for six to 12 months before there is a trial at a lower dose. This lets your child stabilize and return to the level of functioning that was present before the onset of his difficulty or go on to establish a new level of functioning.

At the end of that time, the medication is lowered in small steps, separated by enough time to tell if your child stays stable at the lower dose. The medication continues to be lowered until none is remaining. This is called "tapering" the medication.

If the problem returns after a decrease in the medication, your child then may have the medication raised back up to the earlier dose, for another six to 12 months, before another lowering. If that second trial isn't successful, further trials at lowering the dose might be undertaken after your child has been stable for a whole 12 months.

For some situations in which the symptoms are severe, and going off medication may lead to very worrisome or dangerous behavior, changes are made very slowly. Sometimes your child's doctor may recommend that no changes be considered for several years, especially when there is stress and turbulence expected, as there may be for an adolescent with a serious disorder who is entering high school. In such a situation the use of medication may last until a more stable time is reached in adulthood. Of course, as your adolescent gets older, he takes a more active role in determining whether medication is continued or not. Inevitably the time will arrive when your child has the final say regarding the taking of medication. Therefore, it is essential to involve your child (even at a young age) as much as possible in the decisions made regarding medication. This way, any earlier resentment from feeling excluded and having "no say" about his medication less likely will cloud his decisions about what to do when he is older and has "total say."

5. Will medication continue without psychotherapy?

The short response is yes—medication may continue after the termination of psychotherapy. For example, your child who has attentional problems and has reasonably resolved emotional or behavioral difficulties may continue on medication to maintain a "good enough" level of functioning at school and home. Or, your formerly depressed child may have made major gains in psychotherapy and is doing reasonably well. As part of a plan to end treatment, there is a trial at lowering the medication, but perhaps there is a return of some symptoms. It may be clear that medication should continue for another six to 12 months, but you, your child, and your child's psychotherapist may decide that there are no more important gains to be made from psychotherapy at that point, and medication continues without further therapy.

The longer response is that it is not always so clear cut. For example, you and the therapist may decide to go along with your child's request for a break from therapy since she has been in treatment for quite a while. She has made some modest gains but seems to have hit a plateau and is reluctant to continue. The hope is that after a break, your child, or more often adolescent, will return to psychotherapy. Or the psychotherapy may reach a "stuck point" and ends somewhat abruptly and without plans to continue to try to make gains with another therapist. But medication clearly may be needed and is continued.

Or medication might continue without psychotherapy because an insurance company decides that outpatient psychological treatment will no longer be supported but medication treatment will. If the cost of psychotherapy cannot be borne by your family, your child may continue on medication without psychotherapy until insurance coverage is again available.

Some of these situations are well thought out; others are not. The goal is to make all reasonable efforts so that your child is receiving sufficient and complementary medical and psychological treatments.

Conclusion

Medication can be remarkably helpful, although many times not as helpful as everyone would like. Do not hesitate to raise questions or problems about the medication with your child's doctor.

Psychopharmacology for children is based increasingly on scientific studies, yet is still very much an art and skill. Your child's doctor wants to help. But sometimes the doctor may answer your question about doing more to help your child with "I've tried all that I know how," or "We just don't know enough," and that really may be the case.

When conventional treatment is not enough and parents desire more help, parents may seek alternative forms of treatment. Chapter 10 addresses this topic.

Chapter 10

COMPLEMENTARY AND ALTERNATIVE THERAPIES AND THEIR SIDE EFFECTS

I am often asked about alternative medicinal and non-medicinal treatments—treatments that are not currently mainstream, conventional, or sufficiently supported by evidence-based scientific studies. Some of these treatments are being studied and may enter the mainstream; others are unlikely to. The purpose of this chapter is to describe some common alternative treatments so that you can be more informed making a decision about when, whether, and how to use them.

Organization of Chapter 10

I begin with general comments about the use of non-mainstream forms of treatment. Then I review five common chemical and non-chemical alternative treatments:

- herbal remedies
- vitamin and dietary treatments
- meditation/relaxation training
- neurofeedback
- sensory motor integration therapy.

These alternative treatments are ordered roughly from least to most by how much involvement with a professional each requires. For each category, I address common questions and concerns. I do not address Chinese medicine, acupuncture, or homeopathy except to refer the reader to one of those specialists for more information.

The why, when, and what of alternative treatments

Parents pursue alternative treatments for different reasons.

- They want to treat their child as "naturally" as possible, due to their personal lifestyle or a desire to keep their child free of harmful "artificial" influences.

- They have had unsatisfactory or harmful experiences with the conventional/medical treatment system for themselves, other family members, or their child. These experiences might include pharmacotherapy that was ineffective or produced too many side effects.

- They know a parent who has had success with an alternative treatment for a child with a similar problem.

- They have a child with a medical condition that prevents the child from safely taking certain medications, so they seek non-pharmacological interventions.

- They view complementary and alternative treatments as less intrusive on their parental control and involving less dependency on someone outside the immediate family.

When problems come up, parents are reminded that children's thoughts and feelings are not under their control and a child's behavior is controllable in only a limited fashion and with great effort. Alternative treatments may not challenge a parent's sense of control and independence as much as conventional treatments. For example, herbal treatments and dietary or vitamin supplements may be bought at a local store, with or without expert consultation. A child can learn relaxation breathing and meditation from an expert but then practice at home on his own. Neurofeedback often lasts a short time and usually involves familiar video-type games. And even sensory integration therapy often involves a parent as an active and central participant in providing some of the treatment at home.

Parents may have a child undertake alternative and complementary treatments before, during, or after psychological treatment or medication. Commonly, parents try these treatments before undertaking psychotherapy or pharmacotherapy. Sometimes parents do both at the same time. This is most likely to happen if the parents are disappointed in the progress of current treatment or with the professional helper and cannot talk about it with that person. Parents may also start the treatments simultaneously with the idea that they "want to do everything possible to help my child."

Whatever the reasons for using an alternative treatment, it is important to tell the clinician providing conventional treatment (psychotherapy and especially medication) that your child is undergoing an alternative treatment. Some alternative treatments, such as herbals or supplements, may increase or diminish the benefits or side effects of conventional medications.

Below I describe five common alternative treatments, including any research about their benefits and risks.

Herbal treatment

An herb is a scented annual, biennial, or perennial plant used in medicine or food seasoning. It has a soft stem containing little wood and usually produces seeds. It dies back at the end of the growing season.

Herbs used medicinally affect bodily chemistry and function in ways that have been identified as largely positive by folk and traditional healers. Contemporary scientific studies have in some cases supported these claims and in others have not. It is under investigation which chemicals in the herbs are the active ingredients and the particular ways any positive effects are brought about. It does appear that herbs which affect mood and anxiety do so by affecting the same neurotransmitters that conventional medications alter.

My experience with herbal treatments is limited to infrequent case examples, mostly with adults. In those situations, herbals have at times been helpful. Below I list the herbs that are used most commonly to address emotional and behavioral symptoms.

- *St. John's Wort* is used to treat mild depression.

- *Valerian* is used for sleep.

- *Kava-Kava* is taken for anxiety.

- *Melatonin* (not an herb but a naturally occurring hormone) has been used in a synthetic form as a sleep aid for children. While it is helpful for sleep, some doctors prefer not to recommend a hormone-type medication for regular use by children or teenagers since its long-term impact is not known.

Keep in mind the following when considering herbal treatments:

- There are subtleties to the herbal medications and the prescriptions of them; they need to be individualized to the particular patient and the way that person experiences anxiety, insomnia, worry, depression, etc.

- Especially for children, whose brains are still growing and who react to all sorts of substances ingested in unpredictable and sometimes paradoxical ways, using botanicals for emotional and psychosocial issues should be done only with great caution and understanding.

- Very few botanicals have been tested on children.

- Dosing and frequency of administration for each particular herbal therapy can vary and is best done under professional guidance.

- Responsible professional practitioners of botanical medicine do not practice in a cookbook fashion.

- Discuss the use of herbal treatment with your child's doctor.

- These alternative forms of treatment are still chemical. Do *not* combine them with conventional medications used to address the same symptoms. (For example, do not combine St John's Wort with a conventional antidepressant medication.)

- Although many herbs have been in use for hundreds or thousands of years, they may still produce adverse effects.

- The US government does not regulate the use of herbal preparations as carefully as it regulates the use of pharmaceutical products and unreliable brands exist. So it is hard to determine standard dosages.

All of the remedies below are being studied by the Western scientific community in order to increase understanding of how these medicinals work and the degree to which they are effective.

ST JOHN'S WORT

Use: Treats mild to moderate depression.
Cautions and side effects:

- Do not take with MAOI antidepressants.

- Do not take with selective seratonin reuptake inhibitors (SSRI) antidepressants.

- Do not take with medications for AIDS.

- Do not take with Zyprexia (olanzapine).

- Do not take if pregnant or breast-feeding.

- Use in children should be monitored by a qualified practitioner.

- Women taking St John's Wort occasionally report that their oral contraceptives have failed.

- Side effects include increased sensitivity to sunlight, bloating, and constipation.

- Research has not found many serious side effects. There are potentially dangerous interactions if St John's Wort is used with birth control pills or with medications for organ transplants, thyroid disease, high blood pressure, and high cholesterol.

VALERIAN

Use:

- Treats insomnia (although clinical studies on its effectiveness are inconclusive).

- Used to calm nervousness.

- Sometimes also taken for lack of concentration, headache, premenstrual syndrome, fainting.

Cautions and side effects:

- Has a distinctive stink.
- Do not use with other sedatives or anti-anxiety medications such as benzodiazepines (Xanax, Valium, Klonopin, etc.) listed in Chapter 9, or barbiturates.
- Do not use if pregnant, breast-feeding, or in children under three.
- Can cause digestive problems.
- Long-term use can lead to headache, restlessness, sleeplessness, pupil dilation and heart problems.

KAVA-KAVA

Use: Considered a remedy for anxiety and insomnia.
Cautions and side effects:

- Do not use if pregnant or nursing.
- Can deepen depression; do not use if you have a depressive disorder.
- Do not combine with other drugs/substances that affect the brain (such as alcohol, barbiturates, and mood altering drugs).
- Do not use with children (because of the uncertainty about liver toxicity).
- Do not take for more than three months without medical supervision.
- Use caution when driving.
- Side effects include a tired feeling, upset stomach and gas, loss of balance, pupil dilation, and difficulty focusing.
- High doses of Kava-Kava can trigger hepatitis and liver failure.

MELATONIN

Use: Helpful for insomnia.
Cautions and side effects:

- Do not use with alcohol and tobacco, which interfere with production of melatonin.
- Do not use if depressed.
- Do not use if trying to conceive a child, pregnant, or nursing.
- Caution for use in children or teenagers (see above text).
- Aspirin, beta-blockers, and Inderal decrease melatonin levels, so adjust dosage of melatonin accordingly.

- The SSRI Luvox increases melatonin levels, so adjust dosage of melatonin accordingly.
- Do not combine with Prozac.
- Increases the effect of antihistamines and sedating antidepressants.
- May make you feel tired in the morning when you first take it.
- Use caution while driving.
- Side effects include stomach discomfort, depression, and low body temperature.
- Do not take it for more than two weeks.

Most of the information presented above is cautionary, largely because the use of herbals in young children is unknown as far as conventional medical circles are concerned. Naturopathic doctors, Chinese herbalists, and some chiropractors have extensive experience with these chemicals. Consult with a reputable practitioner if you wish to try these for your child. In addition to following the warnings about combining particular herbals with conventional medications, I again strongly recommend you tell your child's medical doctor or specialist if you are giving herbal therapies to your child.

Vitamin and dietary treatments

For centuries, people have reported that their diet influences their behavior. Therapeutic interventions have involved the following:

- eliminating specific foods
- eliminating artificial flavorings, colorings, or preservatives
- taking dietary supplements
- taking large doses of vitamins and minerals.

Past reports investigating various diets and supplements produced no definitive evidence for a clear effect. But there have been individual reports that limiting sugar or certain processed foods and avoiding artificial coloring, flavoring, or preservatives improved a child's behavior.

I consider such individual observations and reports as valid. And because such interventions often lead to a more healthful diet, I support parents who raise the possibility of trying them even though dietary changes/restrictions may at first generate conflict between parent and child. I support their use as an additional or complementary intervention, but I don't advise them as the primary intervention when a child's symptoms have caused a lot of difficulty and suffering. Diets should not be a substitute when more conventional, often very successful, medication and psychotherapeutic treatment are needed.

Recently some interesting reports and research have made me reconsider my position on how much vitamins and dietary supplements impact behavior and emotions. These reports involve the use of *omega-3 fatty acids, inositol,* and a complex combination of *multi micro-nutrients* (vitamins and minerals). These studies need to be duplicated by more researchers and further investigation is needed to clarify the effectiveness, safety, and best use practices for these supplements. Yet these alternative treatments may offer the possibility for effective, relatively safe and low side effect dietary interventions for some psychiatric disorders. Below, I discuss each of these alternatives and cite articles, numbered and listed at the end of this chapter, for further information.

Omega-3 fatty acids are being studied as a treatment for childhood depression (Nemets *et al.* 2006) with positive results, and there has been a report out of England of a well-run scientific study that suggested benefits for treating childhood attention deficit hyperactivity disorder (ADHD) (Richardson 2006; Richardson and Montgomery 2005). The source for these omega-3 fatty acids used in the study was fish oil, one of the most direct means for providing the EPA and DHA type of omega-3 fatty acid ingredients in the study. While some doctors in practice are recommending these supplements for children with ADHD, no USA researcher has duplicated the study at this point. It appears that a connection between improved behavioral and emotional modulation and these vital dietary building blocks of the nervous system is slowly being made.

Inositol, once thought to be a B vitamin but now seen as more related to glucose, is an active agent in the process of nerve cell transmission. There is some evidence that it is effective in panic disorder (Palatnik *et al.* 2001) and much weaker evidence in depression (Nierenberg *et al.* 2006). However, it may make ADHD and mania worse, usually at excessive doses, beyond the therapeutic range. It does not seem to make the SSRIs more effective, although it has been used to help with sleep problems associated with the SSRIs. Further research to better understand how inositol works and the best ways to use it are needed.

A specific complex of vitamins and minerals, under the trade name *EMpower,* has become a focus of research (Popper 2001). This complex has been reported to be quite helpful for the mood instability of bipolar disorder, and current research is exploring whether it works with statistical reliability. At this point, research doctors do not know which parts of the complex are essential and which incidental or whether all are contributory. Nor do they know how these micro-nutrients work together. The investigators also need to figure out with more detail how to use this complex in combination with more conventional medication, as it can increase a medication's side effects.

The preceding supplements are still in the early stages of study, understanding, and research. I mention them here to highlight that various vitamin and dietary supplements appear to have a valid place in the treatment of behavioral and emotional difficulties.

Meditation and relaxation techniques

Meditation is a state of concentration that involves a focus upon a single, clearly defined object. Frequently that object is the breath, but actually anything may be taken as an object of concentrated attention:

- a sound
- a phrase
- an image
- a bodily sensation.

Formal research has supported meditation's positive effect on the brain and immune function. The practice of meditation can help individuals learn to relax, improve concentration, and cope with stressful emotions or situations. Meditation may also improve *mindfulness*: the ability to be aware of what is happening at the moment and be attentive. Mindfulness, as mindfulness training, is a major component of dialectical behavioral therapy skills training (DBT) (see Chapter 8), and as focal awareness of bodily sensations, it is a central aspect to a newly developed form of psychotherapy called somatic experiencing (SE) therapy which is used for the resolution of post-traumatic stress reactions and symptoms.

"Relaxation techniques" is a term referring to the helpful tools for coping with stress and promoting long-term health by slowing down the body and quieting the mind. Such techniques include *progressive muscle relaxation*, which involves alternatively slowly tensing and releasing each muscle group individually, starting with muscles in the toes and working upwards through the body. *Deep breathing* is another relaxation technique that allows the body to relax itself. Relaxation breathing is an important part of yoga and martial arts for this reason. The technique simply involves taking a number of deep breaths and relaxing your body further with each breath. Another includes *autogenic training*, which is the use of visual imagery and body awareness to enter a state of relaxation through imagining a peaceful place while focusing on the different physical sensations. Also included in the umbrella term, *relaxation techniques*, are the exercises aimed at increased body awareness and connecting mind and body together referred to above—*meditation*.

Commonly, meditation and the various relaxation techniques are added to some types of psychotherapy. Though considered "add-ons," they nevertheless can help address anxiety, sleep disturbances, and the management of intense emotions like anger and fear. Some psychotherapists provide relaxation training and meditation training as a part of treatment. Other therapists may not provide the training but recommend the use of child-focused audiotapes that provide guided imagery, progressive muscle relaxation training, and positive affirmations (see Appendix).

It is easier for a child to learn to use meditation or relaxation techniques when a parent practices along. Parents themselves also benefit from doing meditation and relaxation practices, even if they started just to help their child. Some children, particularly those who like to move their bodies, may find that yoga offers a more acceptable way to get into the practice of breathing/relaxation exercises and meditation.

When used regularly, meditation and breathing/relaxation exercises are very helpful non-medicinal ways to address mild anxiety and sleep difficulties. They may be used safely along with medication for anxiety or mood-related symptoms. Because meditation and breathing/relaxation exercises can lower anxiety, the dose of medication needed to produce a beneficial effect may be lower when used together with these techniques.

Neurofeedback

Neurofeedback, also known as EEG biofeedback or EBF, has been in use clinically since the early 1990s. It is a form of biofeedback, which itself has been used for 40 years and reached wide use in the 1970s. Researchers discovered that humans had more control over bodily functions than previously thought, and biofeedback was used to control blood pressure, muscle tension, and body temperature (autonomic system functions). It is used with positive effect on medical problems such as hypertension and migraine headaches.

As biofeedback teaches an individual to alter blood pressure or muscle tension, so neurofeedback is a technique that teaches an individual how to alter brain wave activity, which is measured by an EEG (electrocephalogram). The theory behind neurofeedback is that the speed and intensity of the brain waves, over different areas of the brain, correspond to different levels of arousal, alertness, and attention. The brain is a complex bioelectrical system. When this system is not working well, we don't feel or function to our full capacity. Depending upon its severity, disruptions in the bioelectrical functioning of our brain can result in:

- problems with focus, attention, and learning
- sleep disruption
- depression, anxiety, and behavioral difficulties
- migraine headaches or seizures.

Neurofeedback training helps a person learn to alter their arousal and alertness to more suitable levels. These changes are associated with positive effects on patterns of thinking and feeling, states of awareness and attention, and ultimately behavior.

Neurofeedback technique uses computer games as the means for engaging the patient in this process. The clinician first determines the particular pattern of brainwave feedback to use, basing this decision on the patient's medical, emotional, and behavioral history. It is also determined by testing that may include a detailed examination of the overall brainwave pattern, called a quantitative EEG analysis, or tests of attention that use computer technology, called a continuous performance test (see Chapter 6 on tests of attentional skill).

Then electrodes are placed on the patient's scalp. This allows for recording and magnification of the EEG or brainwave activity. This brainwave activity is recorded on the clinician's computer, which is also connected to the patient's game computer.

The patient then tries to move some figure in a game on a computer screen. This is done by thinking, breathing slowly, imagining a scene, or even some less conscious activity. The moving object on the screen reflects an increase or decrease in a particular brainwave pattern over a particular area of the brain. The neurofeedback clinician can adjust how much the patient needs to alter the brainwave pattern in order to make the figure on the screen move.

Over a number of sessions, the patient will be able to change to the designated brainwave pattern more easily and increase his brain's ability to shift into a better state of arousal. This better state will help him become more alert, focused, and have better overall operation of his brain's activity, resulting in more balanced emotional states and better daily functioning. With a sufficient number of neurofeedback sessions, the patient will begin to regulate his own brain state spontaneously, resulting in increased positive feeling and functioning.

As the ability to change unwanted states (such as frequent states of poor focus or inattention) becomes more automatic, old, more troublesome patterns are diminished and more effective patterns become established. Neurofeedback helps an individual learn better self-regulation. Improved self-regulation is central to having better influence over one's emotions, behavior, concentration, and attention.

Practitioners of neurofeedback generally report that 65 to 75 per cent of individuals diagnosed with ADHD and treated with this method receive benefit from this intervention in a few sessions, but more sessions are usually needed to sustain the benefits. The number of sessions needed is based upon several criteria:

- the severity of symptoms
- how long the patient has had the problem
- whether or not the patient is taking medications
- how well they stick to the program
- the degree of brain dysfunction.

Some formal studies have found significant gains in the treatment of major behavioral disorders, epilepsy, and sleep disorders. Other studies show no gains.

Generally, insurance companies are reluctant to cover the cost of neurofeedback treatment. Each insurance company has its own criteria for judging the effectiveness of complementary and alternative procedures. Considerably more companies are paying for the treatment presently than there were five years ago. Parents should inquire whether or not their insurance would pay or reimburse for biofeedback rather than neurofeedback. Insurance terminology will include biofeedback, and neurofeedback is a type of biofeedback. Often times parents pay out-of-pocket for treatment. The price ranges from $50–$135 per session, depending upon the experience of the clinician and the geographic location.

Despite current insurance policies, my analysis of the literature indicates that there is enough evidence to support this intervention. I believe that neurofeedback may be helpful in the following circumstances:

- if conventional treatment is inadequate to manage symptoms and there is not more to do

- if there is a wish to increase the effectiveness of medication and perhaps lower the dosage

- if parents are opposed to putting a child on medication and want to try some alternative treatment first.

As we learn more about how the brain and mind work, along with computers and programs becoming even more powerful, I believe a similar method of influencing brainwave patterns will become an important and more widely accepted form of treatment for ADHD and other emotional, behavioral, and learning disorders.

Sensory/motor integration therapy

Sensory integration is based upon the view that the normal way the brain takes in information through the various senses and the way the brain organizes that sensory information can sometimes be quite disrupted. The disruption may occur in the sense of sight, sound, smell, taste, and the modalities of touch (pain, temperature, pressure, and movement). The disruption may happen because a sensory experience is too strong or too weak for an individual child's brain. A child with sensory integration difficulties may have trouble organizing and integrating all or some of the incoming information from the different senses. Symptoms can occur because of this poor integration. A child may experience the following:

- disruptions in walking and other motor movements

- delay in speech development

- problems with attention

- various emotional, behavioral, and learning disorders.

As a child grows older, the brain's ability to integrate sensory experience becomes more sophisticated and complex. Ordinarily, a child's normal play and activity is enough to foster good brain sensory integration.

The theory of sensory integration states that children with *autism*, other serious *developmental disorders*, *learning disabilities*, and *attentional problems* are all more likely to have difficulties with sensory integration. The same is true for children born *prematurely*, exposed to *neglect*, or raised by parents with *substance abuse*. A child whose sensory integration is not age-appropriate may have any of the symptoms mentioned above.

When a child is having difficulties, sensory integration problems may be a central element *or* a complicating factor. Either way, sensory integration treatment may help restore normal brain processing.

Sensory integration therapy (SI) is done by a specially trained occupational therapist one to three times per week. Usually, the therapy takes place in a room with equipment to improve particular sensory experience and foster sensory integration. There may be special swings for improving posture and movement in space, large inflated balls to develop balance, and obstacle courses to enhance motor planning. There may be beanbags to exercise visual–spatial perception and materials of different textures to develop tactile discrimination and decrease tactile defensiveness (avoidance of certain kinds of sensations because of intense discomfort with them).

Parents may work with an occupational therapist to develop a range of activities (called a sensory diet) that can be done at home. Sensory integration may be improved through activities that alert and boost an undersensitive child, activities that calm an oversensitive child and decrease hyper-responsiveness, and activities that specifically help a child organize his sensory experience.

I consider SI "less conventional" because even though many child mental health providers advocate for SI, many still regard the therapy as not sufficiently grounded in definitive research studies. My experience with successful SI therapy is too limited to give my own authoritative conclusion. I support this form of treatment being part of a total treatment program based on the benefits I have seen and the reading I have done. I do not support its use as a substitute when more conventional treatments, such as medication or psychotherapy, are appropriate. (See "The Out of Sync Child" referenced in the Appendix for more information on sensory integration dysfunction.)

* * *

In this chapter I have discussed five treatments considered alternative and complementary to conventional medication and psychotherapy. Please use the resources in the Appendix of the book, and articles cited below, if you wish to explore them further. The next chapter, on play (an expansion of Chapter 8 on psychotherapy), returns to the arena of more conventional therapy and completes the book's material devoted to treatment.

References

Nemets, H., Nemets, B., Apter, A., Bracha, Z. and Belmaker, R.H. (2006) 'Omega-3 treatment of childhood depression: A controlled, double-blind pilot study.' *American Journal of Psychiatry 163*, 1098–1100.

Nierenberg, A.A., Ostacher, M., Calabrese, J., Ketter, T. (2006) 'Treatment-resistant bipolar depression: A STEP-BD equipoise randomized effectiveness trial of antidepressant augmentation with lamotrigine, inositol, or risperidone.' *American Journal of Psychiatry 163*, 210–216.

Palatnik, A., Frolov, K., Fux, M. and Benjamin, J. (2001) 'Double-blind, controlled, crossover trial of inositol versus fluvoxamine for the treatment of panic disorder.' *Journal of Clinical Psychopharmacology 21*, 3, 335–339.

Popper, C.W. (2001) 'Do vitamins or minerals (apart from lithium) have mood-stabilizing effects?' *Journal of Clinical Psychiatry 62*, 12, 933–935.

Richardson, A.J. (2006) 'Omega-3 fatty acids in ADHD and related neurodevelopmental disorders.' *International Review of Psychiatry 18*, 2, 155–172.

Richardson, A.J. and Montgomery, P. (2005) 'The Oxford-Durham Study: A randomized, controlled trial of dietary supplementation with fatty acids in children with developmental coordination disorder.' *Pediatrics 115*, 1360–136.

Stock Kranokitz, C. (1998) *The Out of Sync Child*. New York, NY: Perigee Books.

Chapter 11

THE ROLE OF PLAY
IN INDIVIDUAL PSYCHOTHERAPY
FROM CHILDHOOD TO
ADOLESCENCE

Your image of psychotherapy may be of someone sitting in a chair talking about their feelings and thoughts, a difficult life situation, or a problem relationship. If so, then the idea of bringing your action-oriented seven-year-old son or your tightlipped 14-year-old daughter to psychotherapy may seem odd. But most non-adult patients in psychotherapy do not just sit and talk; they play and talk. The play may take place while sitting at a table, lying on the floor, or standing in front of a basketball hoop. Although play in psychotherapy usually happens inside of an office, it may also take place outside. The play may involve the use of paints or puppets, board games or balls, or just about anything that is used for play. This chapter will help you understand how psychotherapy and play fit together. As you learn more about what goes on in psychotherapy and play therapy, you may feel more at ease taking your child to a stranger for this treatment.

Organization of Chapter 11

Before focusing on play and psychotherapy, I will examine the role of play in your child's job of learning how to manage her body, cope with emotions, engage in relationships and take in information about the world. I will then present a general way of understanding how psychotherapy works: a theory of psychological treatment. This includes a brief discussion about behavior, feelings, and thoughts, and then of memory, a major underpinning for them. I'll discuss change and how it happens: change of memory (called learning) and change of behavior, feelings, and thoughts. Any or all of these may be the focus of the work in psychological treatment.

I then discuss psychodynamic psychotherapy, the specific form of psychological treatment in which play was first used as a part of the therapy process. Next I take a closer look at "play therapy," which uses play as a central means for change and improvement. This section focuses on the practical aspects of play therapy, including the materials used and how a therapy session is organized.

I offer an extended example of one boy's play therapy, so you can see how the play, and the interactions between the therapist and child, helped the boy make positive changes. I end with how you as a parent may fit into your child's play therapy.

Play

Adults know that *play* has an important role in a child's development—as the expression goes, "All work and no play makes Jack a dull boy." But how important is play, and in what ways is it important?

Think about when your child was a baby, long before she was exposed to the common games or other types of play that are part of our culture. You noticed that she played with such things as your hair, her own toes, or a mobile placed over the crib. Her mood was often pleasant or cheerful, and she could usually set aside the play rather easily for some other activity. Your baby was working at the very earliest phases of the jobs of developing a relationship with another person, getting to know and manage her body, and taking in information about the world around her. This occurred as she was experiencing pleasure and joy, emotions which usually go along with the experience of mastery and being in a setting that feels safe.

As your daughter got older, you helped her learn to throw a ball or ride a bike. She then would do that activity over and over, when you were present and when you were not. Usually, a child feels pleasure when she repeats an activity. Through play, your child was learning to manage her body better, interact in a more complex way with another person, and learn even more about the physical world around her. She was also experiencing the pleasure and joy that are part of learning to master an activity and that help her temper or overcome fear.

Play is a complex, vital, and central activity in your child's development from birth to adulthood. Play almost always involves some "work" at problem-solving and mastery. It is an "instrument of learning" that is part novelty (encountering something new) and part repetition (securing what is new). The "stuff" of play usually involves one or more areas of human functioning (see Chapter 3): managing the body, coping with emotions, engaging in relationships, and taking in and processing information about the surrounding world.

A theory of psychotherapy
The complexity underlying feeling, thinking, and behavior

Your child's behavior, feelings, and thoughts—the focus of psychotherapy—are the outcome of at least three factors:

1. the temperament, or nature, that your child was born with
2. the life experiences she has had
3. how those life experiences are organized in her memory.

Temperament refers to the "style" with which your child's nervous system responds and reacts. This can be seen easily in the first month after birth. Most likely you noticed that your child was quite distinctive and different from other babies. She may have reacted quickly, or slowly, to something new that she saw, heard, or felt. Her overall activity level may have been energetic or more laid-back. Her emotional responses might have been strong or mild. These qualities, and many others, are an expression of your child's particular nature or temperamental style.

Life experience includes everything that happened to your child that she could see, hear, taste, smell, and touch/feel: the daily ordinary events and more uncommon and memorable ones. The events of life begin in infancy and last through old age. Early in a person's development the events of life generally seem simpler and more straightforward. With age and more experience comes the ability to make judgments and have expectations. As that happens, the events of life seem more complicated.

The record of your child's life experiences is stored as memory. These life experiences in memory are *organized* and each person has a unique way that what was seen, heard, felt, etc. is stored and put together. How your daughter's life experiences are organized show up in how she remembers an event: its meaning to her. This is a very complex process that is only barely understood.

The relationship between temperament, life experience, and memory organization is extremely complicated. We see small instances of this incredible complexity at work when we notice how the same event may lead to different feelings, thoughts, and behavior within the same person (at different times) or between different people. For example, you might assume that a young child would react with fear if the lights in a room go out suddenly. Yet, sometimes your child might experience the same event of the lights suddenly going out as part of a game; then, she may react more with joy or excitement. Or, as the example below illustrates, one child might react to a friend moving away with anger and protest, while for another child, the same event may result in sadness and withdrawal.

> Seven-year-old Sally was friends with Elizabeth and Sandra. Her father got a job in another state and she sadly left her friends behind as her family moved away.

After Sally left, Elizabeth began to fight frequently with her younger sister. Within a few weeks, she no longer played with her classmate Sandra and began to play with other children.

In contrast, Sandra, an only child, felt sad and moped around after Sally left. She kept asking her mother whether Sally was going to move back and when she could write to her. She was hurt that Elizabeth did not want to play with her any more and needed encouragement from her teacher to seek out other children to play with on the playground.

To summarize: your child's behavior, feelings, and thoughts are shaped and determined by each other and by many other factors: those within her and those acting upon her.

The storage and organization of experience: memory

Your child's memory is the mentally stored record of her life experiences. This includes her basic perceptions: what she saw, heard, tasted, smelled, felt, or touched, at any particular point in her life. It also includes her reactive thoughts and feelings about any particular life experience. Her memory includes both kinds of information, whether the event occurred minutes or years ago.

The content of her memory is stored in her brain and organized in different ways. A simple organization of memory is primarily the sensory experience of an event (i.e. the picture, sound, and other sensations). A more complex organization of memory involves emotional and symbolic connections to the sensory organized memories. This more complex memory seems to be involved in producing the meaning or understanding of an event.

This complex level of memory organization becomes larger and more intricately put together as your child moves from childhood to adulthood. It lets her grow in her ability to make sense of her experience. Her unique organization of memory shapes how she perceives and responds to what is happening around her and to her.

Changes in memory: learning

When the contents of memory are enlarged or changed, we call it "*learning*." We learn in countless ways, both within and outside of our awareness. We learn when we have a new experience or take in new facts and information. And we learn when we think about and reflect upon our past experiences (memories), especially if we're doing that with another person.

Emotion has a complex role in learning. Too much emotion (anger, fear, sadness) seems to interfere with learning: we don't see situations clearly or remember events or facts well when our feelings are wrought up. Too little emotion (boredom or spacey detachment) also does so: we miss a lot of what is happening and memories of events or facts are vague, if even present.

Many opportunities for learning are present in "talking therapy." The ongoing relationship—experiencing and responding to the way the therapist behaves and reacts—is an opportunity to learn. The exposure to new information about behavior, feelings, or thoughts is another opportunity to learn and change. Reviewing old information (memory) and its meaning are other opportunities to learn within the psychotherapeutic process. Which of these opportunities is emphasized will vary from one type of psychotherapy to another.

Learning and psychotherapy

All psychotherapies rely upon taking in new information and enlarging and altering memories as the central process for change. Given that people have many different learning styles and aptitudes, it is no wonder that so many types of psychotherapy exist (see Chapter 8 on different types of psychological treatment).

Some types might focus primarily on your child's own *behavior* and the behavior of others in her life. Other forms focus primarily on your child's *feelings* and *thoughts*. The focus of a particular form of psychotherapy might be on *present* experience, *past* experience, or both. All forms of psychotherapy offer a *relationship* as a means for learning, but some emphasize the relationship itself as a means of learning and change.

A discussion of psychodynamic theory, psychotherapy, and play

One form of psychological treatment, called *psychodynamic psychotherapy*, promotes change (learning) in your child primarily through the medium of the relationship with the therapist. Although the bond formed with the therapist is viewed as central, what is talked about between your child and the therapist is also an essential means for improvement. So, in psychodynamic psychotherapy, learning takes place through the new relationship formed with the therapist and through the new information the therapist offers.

Meaningful learning takes place when emotional experience (feeling) is part of the relationship and is talked about. The focus on your child's feelings about herself and about others is fundamental to the new learning that takes place in psychodynamic psychotherapy. Positive change occurs when your child improves how she copes with the particular feelings and deeper emotions that are central to the problems that brought her to treatment.

Many different types of psychodynamic theories explain the effectiveness of psychodynamic psychotherapy. In the material below I present some ideas, common to all the different theories, which will help you understand why psychodynamic psychotherapy emphasizes relationships and feelings, and how change takes place in this process.

Psychodynamic theories of the mind

The term *mind* refers to the invisible organization that underlies human feeling, thinking, and behavior. This organization is invisible not only from the outside by others, but is also largely invisible from the "inside": it is not conscious. Generally speaking, psychodynamic theories share this view that the human mind is largely unconscious.

This complex organization of mental functioning referred to as the *mind* is contrasted with the *brain*. The brain is the visible, complex, material basis of mental functioning. We can see the brain through various techniques used by neuroscientists, who explore the brain's chemical and electrical properties as well as its parts and connecting pathways. The more we learn about the brain, the more we can marvel at the organization of the mind. Although we know that brain and mind are intimately related, the details of that relationship are likely to be a mystery for a long time.

The mind is thought to be composed of subsystems that interact and result in organized behavior and conscious thoughts, images, and feelings. Different theories propose different types of subsystems, or levels, of organization. These theories originally came about because psychiatrists and psychologists were trying to make sense of the complexity, consistency, and changeableness of human feeling, thinking, and behavior. Much of the richness and depth of human mental functioning, which generates emotions, thoughts, and action, grows out of our capacity to find and create extremely intricate patterns in the world around us and within us. Our nature as human beings grows out of our ability to organize experience with emotion, meaning, and symbolism.

Various psychodynamic theories share a *developmental perspective* which suggests a view that there is a continual process of growth and change that takes place in the mind throughout a human life. Learning is possible from infancy through old age. A developmental perspective (see Chapter 3) has several other implications:

1. Children are not little adults.

2. There is a difference between the mental organization of a child (more emotional factors) and that of a developed adult (more rational factors).

3. Both types of organization (more emotional/child and more rational/adult) exist in a state of tension in all adults.

4. The balance in this state of tension is naturally changeable. In response to internal and external stress, the mind can move in the direction of more constructive organization or less constructive organization.

5. Everyone needs positive assistance from others to foster and maintain our highest level of constructive mental organization.

Psychodynamic theories also share the view that certain *human experiences* have a powerful impact upon the organization of the mind. Primary among such experiences are *human relationships*. When a relationship increases feelings of safety, goodness, specialness, and confidence, and decreases feelings of pain, fear, badness, worthlessness, and incompetence, it is experienced as compassionate and meaningful. Over time in such a relationship, different qualities of mental organization that are positive and stable are created—qualities like trust, flexibility, hopefulness, and confidence. These qualities seem to be associated with the view that experience "makes sense" and has "meaning." Behavior that grows from such a view makes sense to others and takes others' feelings and needs into account. On balance, caring and compassionate relationships early in life have a positive impact on the quality of mental organization. This positive influence can continue to exist well into adult life, independent of other life experiences.

Since relationships are imperfect, there are also times in all relationships when feelings of safety, goodness, specialness, and competence are decreased and feelings of pain, fear, badness, and worthlessness are increased. Negative and unstable qualities of mental organization are created. This includes mistrust, rigidity, pessimism, and doubt. These qualities foster the view that our experience is "senseless" and "without meaning." Behavior that grows from such a view seems senseless to others and excessively self-centered.

Losses and separations are other types of important and meaningful life experience that impact upon mental organization. At the simplest level of experience are the small everyday-loss incidents of change, disappointment, and frustration. Examples include your daughter's experience of her friend canceling their movie date or your son's response to his piggy bank having less money in it than he had thought. Such experiences result in adjustments in your child's mental "map" of how the world works. An important part of this change in mental organization involves changes in how the emotions that go along with experiences of loss and separation are managed or soothed. As your child develops, such emotions become less intense, less abrupt, and more composed.

If your child is fortunate, the major losses and changes that are also part of life experience may occur infrequently in her early life. Examples of emotionally stressful events include the challenges of serious medical or psychiatric illness or the major disruptions in caring and compassionate relationships due to divorce or abuse. The ultimate experience of separation and loss is with death. Such major losses normally result in significant mental reorganization of the images of self and others. Sometimes the reorganization results in a mental life that is wiser, emotionally better adjusted, and more resilient. At other times the reorganization results in a mental life that is more confused, emotionally unsettled, and vulnerable.

Included in this process of mental change are the adjustments of your child's inner images of herself and other people. When a child is young, these images are usually in the extreme, either positive or negative. In response to what is learned from experience and an improved ability to handle emotions, these images become more realistic and less extreme. That is, the images of self and others become more reasonable. With more stable emotions and more realistic images of self and others, a child increasingly develops a sense of resilience in the face of separations and loss.

There are many other important life experiences that influence mental organization. This includes experiences that are part of *normal physical and social development*. For example, as your child moves into puberty, his childhood mental organization undergoes a major reorganization. These major alterations in the mind are driven by hormonal increases, body and brain growth, and changed social expectations. Later stages of life such as marriage, parenthood, and physical aging also result in substantial mental reorganization, especially the images of self and others. Again, the reorganization sometimes results in a mental life that is wiser and emotionally better adjusted; other times it results in a mental life that is more confused and emotionally unsettled.

A theory of psychodynamic psychotherapy

From the perspective of the theory just discussed, we can better understand how psychodynamic psychotherapy is helpful. Through the relationship and what is talked about, some particular aspects of mental organization (mind) are altered in a positive direction. This may have to do with self-image, relationships with others, the experience of loss and separation, or how particular emotions are handled. This positive alteration may help particular ideas, images, expectations, etc. become less fantastic and more realistic, less immature and distorted, less erratic and unsettled, and more steady and integrated. Through psychodynamic psychotherapy the images of self, others, and the world can become more connected to comforting positive emotions and less connected to disturbing negative emotions.

The sources for such positive change in your child's mind may result from the two means for learning in psychodynamic psychotherapy: the *relationship* between your child and the therapist, and the *communication* that takes place between them. These two ways of learning are distinct but mutually interactive. The quality of the relationship influences how the communications are interpreted, and the communications influence the quality of the relationship.

The experience of a positive and helpful new *relationship* with a therapist is an extremely important force for constructive change in your child's feelings, thoughts, and behavior. Developing this kind of therapeutic relationship takes time. It begins with the experience of the therapy setting as a friendly, comfortable, and safe place. Such feelings can be helped along through the use of toys and other objects of play. As the setting feels more friendly and safe, your child can begin to experience the therapist as caring and interested. Through regularly scheduled meetings, your child has the chance to experience the therapist as understanding. Your child comes to feel that she is cared about, is interesting and understood, and her mood and sense of self become more positive. Within the sessions, your child might begin experiencing better ways for handling her feelings, of thinking about the people and events in her life, and of interacting with others. Her more positive state of feeling, thinking, and interacting usually differs from how your child was when she first came to therapy. If strong enough, such positive states and the related change can carry over to her home and school life.

With an increased sense of safety and being understood, and decrease in anxiety, your child is more able to take in and benefit from the second means for positive change: the therapist's *communications*. These communications can be primarily *verbal* (relying upon language) or *non-verbal*. In either case, the ultimate goal is to help your child make sense of, and cope better with, whatever difficulty brought her to therapy. The difficulty might be a specific event (such as a very ill parent, a divorce, or the birth of a sibling). Or it might be not a particular event, but rather one of a number of specific challenging life experiences (such as coping with ordinary separations, playing with other children, or managing feelings of anger, fear, or disappointment). Some children seem to weather such events with minimal disruption; others find such life experiences very challenging.

In therapy that has little play, the therapist's *verbal communications* will be comments, questions, and observations in response to what your child says. In play therapy the therapist's verbal communications include comments about the action going on in the play. The therapist's *verbal communications* might be making a comment on a game board move, noting what an animal figure is doing, or describing what is being drawn. Or he may comment on the emotions or motivations expressed in the play. For example, the therapist may note how alone or sad a figure in a drawing looked, or may wonder why the toy horse was burying itself in the sand. The therapist's tone is generally one of understanding and acceptance, as well as gentle curiosity.

At a point that seems tactful, the therapist may comment about the content of the play and its relationship to the current problem that brought your child to treatment. Such *verbal communications* grow out of the understanding of your child that the therapist has gained from their interaction. It also comes from discussions with you. One aim of these verbal exchanges is to help your child understand and accept emotional experience (her own and others').

The *non-verbal communications* within psychodynamic psychotherapy are harder to identify but are very important in promoting a sense of acceptance and understanding between your child and her therapist. Non-verbal communication may be expressed as a shrug, a nod, a smile, a sigh, or through how much the therapist lets your child determine what activities are engaged in, how much the therapist participates in the play, and the quality of the emotional energy the therapist brings to the play.

Whether verbal or non-verbal, the back and forth communications between your child and her therapist contribute to a gradual change in her mental organization. As talk and play takes place and the relationship between them becomes more secure and communicative, your child's sense of herself and her mood become more positive. In response to the therapist's communications, further new learning—about the difficult situation she has to deal with or the emotions she experiences—takes place in your child. New learning means your child has some new organization in her mind which shows up as changes in her feelings, thoughts, and behavior. These changes signal an improved capacity to cope with her emotions and the particular situation that led to therapy. An improved capacity to cope generally also means a decrease in her worrisome symptoms.

Put another way, through the back and forth of these communications, your child can come to know and trust her therapist more fully. When this happens, your daughter brings up more intensely personal and troubling emotional experience, either directly through talking or within the play. By intensely personal, I mean emotional experience important to her sense of security and safety. By troubling, I mean an experience (usually a loss or separation) that involves emotions such as fear, anger, disappointment, guilt, and shame.

Each child starts therapy at a different level of *trust*, which reflects her view of how much she can depend upon the therapist to help her and not hurt her. The level of trust also reflects the strength of the positive and negative qualities of the images of her parents and other adult authority figures in her mind. Her level of trust also indicates how much disappointment and hurt she imagines she can tolerate without feeling overwhelmed. This, of course, reflects certain qualities of her self-image that exist in her mind. With the development of deeper trust, your child is more open to the observations, suggestions, and understanding that the therapist offers.

Both your child and the therapist contribute to the development of deeper trust. The level of trust may be seen in the ease and spontaneity with which talk and play takes place. When difficulties arise in a trusting relationship, a child and therapist can talk directly about them. And they can also talk about the feelings that are part of the difficulty and differences, especially from the child's viewpoint. This kind of communication is an opportunity for your child to develop a richer understanding and acceptance of her own emotional experience and that of another person. Such deeper understanding and acceptance reflects a positive change in your child's mental organization and also makes further positive change more possible. When this happens, it shows up in positive changes in her external behavior.

Psychodynamic psychotherapy and play

"But," you may wonder, "what if my child doesn't have such developed language ability, or won't use it, and therefore can't talk directly about such complicated experiences as feelings towards her parents, sibling, or teacher?"

Language is not the only way to communicate. Experience is itself symbolically organized in the mind and can be communicated through *play* (perhaps through drawing, small figure play, or in interactive games) through which your child represents what is troublesome in her life and inside her.

Remember, when your child develops symptoms, she is having trouble with one or another aspect of her job: managing her body, coping with her emotions, engaging in relationships, and taking in information about the world. Although she cannot talk about these problems, she can "play about them." The therapist's task is to find effective means for your child to communicate her difficulties symbolically through the play.

In fact, a child frequently comes to therapy because the capacity to play out difficulties has been disrupted or not sufficiently developed. When that capacity to play is blocked, a child misses out on a wonderful skill for discovering good resolutions to problems. Through the use of play ability already there, or an improved capacity to play with the help of the therapist, your child can discover better solutions to problems, and develop more effective internal methods for coping with the troubling emotions that led to treatment. Armed with these gains, she can get "back on track" with her job.

The extended example below illustrates how interactions during play therapy helped one young boy begin to make sense of his vulnerability and his anger. In parentheses, I describe how the therapy progressed, commenting on how the therapist's actions, and the play itself, helped these positive changes take place.

Roger was a bright seven-year-old little boy who liked to build complex structures with whatever materials were at hand. He did well in school except for the fact that when he encountered frustration, he had major tantrums that included cursing, screaming, hitting, kicking, and biting anyone nearby. As a consequence, he had no friends.

Roger's parents had divorced when he was two years old. He had no siblings. His mother, his primary caretaker, frequently felt physically and emotionally overwhelmed caring for her small child and would loudly yell at Roger whenever he did something she didn't want him to do. Roger's father had little to do with his son; occasionally he sent him a birthday card and gift.

Roger spent the first couple of months in therapy building complex structures with the blocks and Legos that were in his therapist's office. (Roger was very cautious about letting any meaningful emotion arise, as his level of trust was quite low.) While initially he protested going to therapy, he gradually began to voice his interest and eagerness about going to sessions and working on a particularly complex structure that he was building with the therapist over the course of many weeks. (The setting and therapist began to seem safer and Roger became more relaxed and comfortable in the sessions.)

Within the meetings, he gradually became less quiet and cautious and more chatty and playful. (Gradually he is developing more trust.) All of this centered on his play and never on his life with his mother, problems at school, or the absence of his father.

At one point he grabbed a toy baby bottle and began sucking on it while he built his structures. He seemed to watch the therapist closely for some critical or belittling comment. There was none, and he began to suck on it regularly. (Roger takes a chance and comforts himself in a desirable and self-satisfying manner that appears to be associated with feelings of shame and fear.) One day he filled the bottle with water and began using baby talk with the therapist. (Roger increases his level of trust in himself and the therapist and lets them both see and be more accepting of his vulnerable and dependent sides. He is symbolically playing out how much he feels like a needy baby.) Outside the sessions, his tantrums became less frequent. (His growth in his sense of acceptance and a more positive sense of self are reflected outside the session.)

Over the following year, Roger incorporated animal play figures into his building projects. (Symbolically, Roger lets more emotional material enter into his play.) There was a skunk that was very angry and nobody liked "because he smelled," and a dinosaur that was orphaned and "always hungry." A repetitive scenario evolved with these figures: the skunk was excluded from the buildings and being with the other animals because he smelled and the dinosaur would devour and destroy the buildings because he could never get enough to eat. (Roger symbolically explores different self-images as expressed in the play characters.)

The therapist emotionally played out and elaborated on his assigned roles as skunk, dinosaur, or other animals under the direction of Roger. (The therapist puts words to unidentified emotions and feelings that go along with these different self-images/animals. For example, it evolved in the play that the skunk only smelled when he got angry, which happened when he was frightened and sad, particularly at times when nobody seemed to want to play with him. When he agreed to not angrily spray the other animals, it turned out they were more likely to let him play.)

Roger's use of the baby bottle and infantile speech within the session diminished and eventually disappeared. (He develops other ways to organize and address his need to comfort himself that are more age-appropriate.) With tantrums occurring less often at home and in school, Roger began to play with other children. A positive spiral of improved tolerance for frustration and improved relationships with others, most importantly his mother, ultimately led to the ending of therapy, even though his particular difficulties were never explicitly talked about.

Practical aspects of play therapy

In the preceding section I described how play is used in therapy to build a relationship and as a vehicle for change. I now focus on the *practical aspects of play therapy*, as it is used with a child from toddlerhood to about age 11 or 12. I describe the setup of a playroom and provide more examples of how play therapy is used as a tool to bring emotional problems to light and address them.

The playroom: Typically, play takes place in a room set up to allow freedom of movement without concern that something will be broken. The space has different kinds of materials depending upon the age of your child, the types of problems that led to therapy, the office setting, and the comfort of the therapist.

Commonly there are objects used for creating two-dimensional images (pencils, markers, crayons, paints, etc.) and some for creating three-dimensional images (clay, Legos, building blocks). There may be small figures that can be manipulated (animals, human dollhouse figures, puppets) and used for creating action stories on the floor, on the table, in a sandbox, or at a water table. Objects that can be used for life-size fantasy play such as telephones, dolls, tea sets, dress-up clothes, or toy weapons might be in the playroom also. In general, the setting resembles a well-stocked play area in a kindergarten or grade-school classroom. For older children, the stock of props might include "tabletop" games or large muscle games, like a basketball hoop or a wiffle bat and ball. As the therapist gets to know your child, there may be an opportunity to bring in some play material specific to your child (like a model building kit). These different play objects can be used by the child alone or in interaction with the therapist.

Before the first session: Before seeing your child, the therapist will probably talk with you. He might suggest how to prepare your child for her first meeting with the therapist. Most likely that meeting, especially for a non-adolescent, will take place in the playroom. The therapist may encourage you to tell your child that you have met with the therapist and that it is okay to talk about personal matters. You might add that you are talking with the therapist to figure out how you can help things improve for your child with regard to her symptoms. Such preparation can reduce the fear and shame that children often feel when they talk with a stranger about personal matters.

The first session: At the first meeting, the therapist will introduce himself and invite your child to check out the playroom. He might be quiet and see how your child responds, or he might encourage her by saying that she is welcome to do what interests her. Depending upon your child's age, as well as her temperament, level of anxiety or depression, and comfort with adults, she will begin to engage with the therapist in her characteristic manner. She may be shy and quiet or be very active and chatty; she may engage in some very imaginative play with small figures, pursue some solitary activity, or offer to toss a ball back and forth.

At some tactful point, after noting that your child's initial anxiety has lessened, the therapist may comment about why she came to therapy. He may say that this first meeting is one of a few in which he will try to learn more about her view of the problem for which her parents brought her there. Or he may indicate that this is the beginning of their spending regular time together, playing and talking, to help her with her problem and feelings. He might be specific about the kinds of feelings she is having trouble with and the circumstances in which the difficulties appear. For example, he may empathically acknowledge her angry feelings towards her baby brother, or sad feelings about her (absent) father, or how painfully shy and embarrassed she gets with grown-ups, peers, or new acquaintances. The emphasis is on emotions and relationships.

It varies as to how long it will take your child to engage in the play and use it to help herself. From the beginning, she may experience the therapist as an adult who offers her a safe and secure setting in which to play in such a way that she is able to get "back on track." Or, it may take her a while. She may be like some children who need help in developing a secure and safe attachment to the therapist or in using play to work out some difficulty. The therapist may initiate the play himself and work to engage your daughter in the play so as to demonstrate its usefulness and encourage her to join in. For example, he may actively participate in small figure play, help develop stories, or encourage some new kind of play. The example below illustrates how the sense of safety gradually developed between me (the therapist) and one young boy.

> Frankie, an eight-year-old boy who had been having prolonged and frequent temper tantrums, came into my office and noted the large dollhouse, family figures and furniture. He commented with disdain that he would never play with that "stuff" because it was "girls' play." I commented that while that might have been his experience, I had found that many boys found the dollhouse rather interesting. Over the course of the next few weeks he "lingered" more and more at the dollhouse, introducing a variety of wild animals and other figures and turning it into a "jungle house." He eventually spent a lot of time symbolically playing out important family experiences that were frightening and overwhelming to him. Gradually his temper tantrums diminished in intensity and eventually disappeared.

Comments that link the play to the child's experiences outside of the office: In the normal course of play therapy, your child's therapist comments about the play as it happens in the office. But early in treatment, the therapist will rarely make comments that link difficulties and events outside the office to the play in the office. This is because if very strong emotions are raised, the flow of play may be disrupted. Only when it seems that your daughter feels safe enough will the therapist sensitively bring up the potentially embarrassing and distressing "outside difficulties." The following story illustrates how I gradually began to comment on connections between the play and one young boy's difficulties with peers at school.

> Juan was a 12-year-old boy who had significant difficulties getting along with peers and making friends. He wanted to spend most of the time in therapy playing board games or engaged in other competitive activities. It wasn't long before it became clear that it was extremely important for him to win these games, so much so that he often cheated, even when he was ahead! As you might imagine, this cheating was a central factor in his peer problems.
>
> My first comments were about our play. I somewhat lightheartedly talked about how I was gradually realizing that he was setting up "special rules" that we were to play by and how surprised I was to find that out, since he hadn't told me. My comments and our discussion remained focused on our relationship and play together for a long period of time. I thought that if I made a link between this behavior with me and his outside problem before he felt safe enough with me, he might feel too humiliated and angry to become more trusting. If that were to

happen, any other observations or understanding I might bring to his difficulty would "fall on deaf ears."

Over many months we worked on the interaction between us, including his need to win, and his feelings of failure and worthlessness. Gradually his fear of losing underlying the pressure to win decreased and his need for "special rules" with me lessened. We increasingly spent time talking about the details of his relationship problems outside the session and he began to have more success making and keeping friends.

Parents and play therapy

Change takes time. Even if you understand the theory and practice of play therapy, it can be hard for you as a parent to bring your child to weekly therapy. If you don't notice any change for quite a while, you will wonder about the value of the time spent in play. Change can be slow. It takes time for a child to build a trusting relationship so that meaningful topics can be addressed, just as it does for an adult. It usually will take at least 20 or more weekly meetings (five months) to build the relationship and begin to see change happen.

As a parent, you are eager to see change as soon as possible: you are worried about your child and also about the financial pressures. Treatment costs money. Managed care arrangements often provide only a limited number of sessions.

To counterbalance some of this pressure you can feel, it is important to develop a trusting relationship with the therapist. A parent–therapist alliance is built over time through frequent meetings that address your worries and concerns as well as your child's struggles. A good relationship with the therapist helps counter a common parental fear that the therapist will become "too important" to the child and somehow take over the role of parent. Meetings with the therapist can help you develop a new perspective on your child, raise questions, discuss your uncertainties, and think about new ways to deal with difficult parenting situations.

If after four to six months of play therapy you notice minimal or no improvement, raise your concerns with your child's therapist. He most likely has similar concerns. Do *not* just drop out of therapy altogether. Instead, consider alternative or additional interventions, or have a consultation with another professional to address some of the following circumstances that might be present.

Your child may be too anxious, depressed, or guarded to feel safe enough with the therapist to engage in play that allows a trusting relationship to develop, even after many meetings. Your child's attention span and hyperactivity level may interfere with her ability to settle into using play constructively enough to address problems. Instead, she may use the meetings more for motor and tension discharge. Your child may be too emotionally "raw" and sessions lead to too much anger, sadness, or shame. In such situations, it is appropriate to consult with a child psychiatrist to consider medication.

Your child may not make progress in therapy because the external stressors in her life are too immediate and too great. Examples of external hindrances to improvement include major parental strife that continues while your child is in therapy, any other situation at home or in school in which your child feels persistently unsafe, or a view on your child's part that certain "secrets" cannot be shared with anyone.

Another reason therapy may not be going as well as hoped might be that the *match* between the therapist and your child isn't right. There may be a large personality or style difference, or the gender match doesn't work. Or your child feels unfairly singled out by others as "the problem," believing herself that the difficulties are contributed to by others in the family. A barrier to work occurs because engaging fully in the therapy might seem to acknowledge that the difficulties are "all her fault." If such circumstances are present, family therapy may be added to the individual sessions.

In other situations, a child's entry into play therapy seems to work like magic. Your child is eager to go to therapy, talks about her therapist frequently, and seems upbeat. Dramatic changes seem to have taken place in a short period of time. You may feel delighted with the relief brought by improvement, somewhat dejected that this "stranger" seems to bring about changes so quickly, or both. Keep in mind that "placebo" responses take place not only with medication. Your child may be attributing special, even fantastical, power to the therapist. This may bolster her self-esteem or reduce her sense of vulnerability and inadequacy.

Do not stop therapy abruptly in the face of such sudden improvement. It may lead to the quick return or increase of her symptoms. Talk about your observations with your child's therapist. The therapist may see such a response as a preliminary phase in the work of forming a trusting relationship that can tolerate difficult emotions or topics that will come up later. Such "idealization" of the therapist by your daughter generally tempers over time. There are situations in which such views of the therapist allow a child to take chances in the real world that she could not do otherwise, and real positive change then can take place.

I hope that this chapter helps you better understand the use of play in psychotherapy and how and why it is so central in play therapy. In retrospect, parents usually feel that change and gains that have happened through play therapy were well worth the financial, emotional, and time "costs" that were involved in supporting the treatment. You will find more about these costs in Chapter 12.

Chapter 12

COSTS OF TREATMENT: MONEY, ENERGY, AND TIME

Raising and caring for your child has many costs, financial and otherwise. Given the present-day financial costs of mental health care, and the daily demands on parents' emotional and time resources, it's no wonder that providing proper treatment for a child can be a major challenge for parents. I hope the material in this chapter prepares you for the anticipated and unanticipated costs of having your child in treatment. Knowing about these different costs can help you prepare to meet the outlay of money, energy, and time associated with getting the professional treatment needed to help your child or adolescent get back on track.

Organization of Chapter 12

I focus first on the financial costs of treatment with different specialists and with various medications (when not covered by insurance).

I then examine the other kinds of costs involved in treatment: your emotional energy and time. These are mainly connected to the treatment experience, but also to dealing with the insurance and managed care companies.

I end with attention to the costs of *non*-treatment—of doing nothing. These costs are harder to calculate. I look at this issue from the perspective of a parent with a child needing treatment and of a tax-paying member of society in which many children need treatment.

Your financial costs for treatment

Below, I concentrate primarily on out-of-pocket costs for psychotherapy and medication: the costs if you do not have insurance coverage. Even if you have health insurance, there may be major gaps in your coverage with regard to mental health coverage. Or, you may choose a clinician who is not covered by your insurance or seek treatment beyond the time limits provided by your managed care coverage.

The financial costs of psychotherapy

Professional treatment may be a crucial component of getting your child back on track. The cost of such care varies widely. Table 12.1 outlines cost for treatment with various specialists.

Your insurance may cover most of the cost of a limited number of sessions with a specialist. But you and the clinician may decide that your child needs a longer term of treatment. You may then have to pay for treatment yourself, referred to as "out of pocket."

Sometimes clinicians will accept fees lower than the listed rates if the client is paying out of pocket to make it more possible to continue treatment when the insurance coverage ends or simply to free themselves from insurance company pressure and oversight.

In a *market economy*, health care fees are set by the same forces that set fees for other services. One force is *supply and demand*. If the number of clinicians stays the same, and more people seek treatment, then prices will go up. If more clinicians are competing to provide services, then prices will go down. Managed care companies keep their cost down by having only a few positions available on the company list of approved providers for clinicians in any one area. Clinicians must compete for those positions, which means that in order to get on the list they agree to accept a lower reimbursement fee than had been their "going rate." A clinician associated with an insurance company will get many referrals but must accept its fee. Because there may be fewer clinicians

Table 12.1 Private or clinic cost of psychotherapy (sliding scale not included)

Type of specialist	Cost of session	Comments
Child psychiatrist: individual or parent counseling session	$100–250 (45–50 minutes)	Cost depends on your geographic location and training/experience of psychiatrist
Psychologist: individual or parent counseling session	$80–150 (45–50 minutes)	Cost depends upon your geographic location and extent of testing
Psychological testing	$400–$2000+	
Clinical social worker: individual or parent counseling session	$40–100 (45–50 minutes)	Cost depends on your geographic location and training/experience of clinician
Any specialist: group therapy	$20–40 (60–90 minutes)	Cost variation depends on your geographic location, specialist, and group length

than needed providing a service for a particular managed-care company, parents who need a therapist for their child might find it hard to locate someone with an opening.

Another market force is the *skill and training* required for the particular service provided. If a service or task requires more skill and training, then the price is higher. That is why clinicians at a doctorate level (MDs and PhDs) are paid more than clinicians at the masters level. This is true even if clinicians at two different levels of training do the same task, for example psychotherapy: people expect that those with more training are more knowledgeable and skilled.

A third market force is the *value of the service* assessed by the clinician providing the service and the person receiving it. This element "fine-tunes" the factors of supply and demand. For example, a particular clinician may be considered especially skilled and may charge more than other similarly trained/qualified clinicians. However, insurance companies consider all individuals with the same level of training to be equal in skill and pay all of them the same.

A *sliding fee scale* is sometimes available to reduce the expected cost of treatment. A sliding scale means that the charge a person pays for a service is based upon their ability to pay. Some private clinicians provide sliding scale fees and others do not. Almost all public clinics use a sliding scale for the cost of psychotherapy. Unfortunately, public funding (from local, state, or federal government) for outpatient clinics has gone down, so the sliding scale doesn't slide to as low a minimum payment as it used to.

The financial costs of medications

As mentioned in Chapter 8, often medication and psychotherapy are *both* required to help your child adequately. Each treatment addresses your child's troubles in a different way.

Medications are generally expensive, and several factors contribute to the high cost. First, many of the medications in common use are new, and are thus available only in the more expensive *brand-name* version. Patents protect these newly created medications for many years: only the company that formulated the drug is allowed to produce it, and that company sets the price. *Generic medication*, available after the patent wears off, is less expensive than brand-name medication because many competing pharmacies make a particular medication.

A second factor that can contribute to the high cost of medication is that generally your psychiatrist thinks first about what medication is best for your child, not what is least expensive. Often the very best medication treatment available to the particular problem your child is having is a new medication which does not yet have a generic form available.

Many insurance companies and state supported programs try to limit doctors to using only generic medications, requiring extra paperwork to justify using the more costly "brand-name" medication. This paperwork, and the delay it takes to wait for a response, discourage the use of the "brand-name" medication. As a result, many doctors have begun to think more about the cost of a medication when making treatment choices and not simply about prescribing "the very best" medication from an effectiveness perspective.

If you don't have prescription coverage and must personally pay for the whole cost of the medication, tell your doctor. He may be able to factor this in when choosing a medication for your child, while still providing good treatment. Yet sometimes, after considering the pros and cons of different medications, you and the doctor will agree that only a brand-name medication will do. If so, ask about your child's eligibility for pharmaceutical company programs that provide medication free of charge for qualifying patients.

In Table 12.2 I list the *approximate monthly cost* for different types of medications, taken at an average dose. It may help you to compare these costs to other more optional expenses in your budget. For example, going to a movie four times a month costs about $28–$36, smoking one pack a day of cigarettes for a month costs about $115, and drinking two bottles of domestic beer a night for one month costs $30–$60.

Note that the medication price may vary widely, depending on whether the medication is generic or brand name.

Table 12.2 Brand-name and generic costs of various psychiatric medications

Medication type examples	Approximate monthly cost for name-brand	Approximate monthly cost for generic
Stimulant medications		
Ritalin	$25–35	$13–20
Concerta	$80–100	not yet available
Adderall	$55–110	$40–80
Antidepressant medications		
Prozac	$80–160	$7–60
Zoloft	$75–150	not yet available
Lexapro	$60–80	not yet available
Mood stabilizers		
Lithium	$60–120	$15–30
Depakote	$125–150	$60
Antipsychotic medications		
Haldol	$75–150	$2.50–$5
Risperidal	$150–300	not yet available
Zyprexa	$240–360	not yet available

Insurance co-pay charges for medications (which vary from insurance plan to insurance plan) are considerably less than the above out-of-pocket costs. Nevertheless, most people are taken aback by the high dollar cost of some of the brand-name psychiatric medications. Unfortunately this high cost can often lead to financially strapped parents prematurely stopping medication, even though they would agree that money spent to help a child feel and function better is money well spent.

As the next section shows, the costs of treatment are not limited to just the financial.

Your energy and time costs in treatment

There are two main non-monetary costs to having your child in treatment:

- emotional energy costs
- time costs.

Your *emotional energy costs* begin even before you start treatment, as you come to grips with the fact that your child has a problem with which you need professional help. When therapy starts, you expend emotional energy opening yourself to a stranger and sharing private family experience. During treatment, you expend emotional energy in the psychotherapeutic work itself (whether in parent, family, couple, or group therapy). You might feel quite energized, especially as you begin to feel the positive effects of the psychotherapeutic work. But at times you might also feel quite depleted.

If your child or some other member of the family resists therapy, you will have an increase in emotional expenses as you support, encourage, and tolerate their fear, anger, shame, and other distressing feelings. Fortunately, your therapist can help with these situations. When such issues are addressed, your emotional costs can be reduced.

Your *time costs* begin when you start trying to figure out where to go for services. Two things will save you time:

- Call the specific mental health services number on the back of your insurance card, rather than the main medical insurance number (many insurance companies have a special division in charge of mental health).

- Get the names of mental health providers from a pediatrician who knows your health coverage and the local providers. This will save you from finding out later that some of the providers listed by the managed care staff no longer provide services through your insurance company.

Time costs continue once treatment has begun. You will spend hours going to sessions and driving to and from those sessions. If more than one meeting is scheduled per week (which often happens at the start of treatment), you may feel that the time costs outweigh the benefits of treatment. More than likely, this skeptical view is an expression of your frustration and disappointment at having to deal with your child having difficulties and needing treatment to address them. Take the long-term practical view: the time spent getting treatment for your child is probably far less than the time you would have to spend worrying about and attending to the consequences of unaddressed difficulties.

This brings us to the last topic: not getting the needed treatment for your child.

Costs for non-treatment: personal and community perspectives

All chosen paths have drawbacks and benefits. There are costs for non-treatment (at both the personal and societal level) just as there are costs for treatment.

Personal costs of non-treatment

At first, you may not see the personal costs of non-treatment for emotional and behavioral problems. It might look like: no treatment = no outlay of money. But the *financial costs of non-treatment* add up:

- It costs money to replace property that's destroyed during angry outbursts.
- It costs money to replace money that your child steals for impulsive buying, gambling, or substance usage.

The same is true for the *time costs of non-treatment*:

- You lose time from work if you have to go to recurrent meetings with school staff to discuss attendance or performance problems.
- You lose time at the doctor's if your child has physical complaints that have an emotional basis.
- You lose time if you have to go to court because your child is acting out in the community.

The *emotional costs of non-treatment* vary, but are always there:

- You, your family, and your child may have years of emotional suffering and unhappiness if your child does not get treatment.
- You may experience high levels of ongoing worry, guilt, anger, sadness, and emotional turbulence within the family.
- Your child's brothers/sisters may have to bear the emotional costs of an untreated impaired sibling well into their own adult lives. Early proper treatment can make huge differences in the future emotional lives of all family members.

The decision to enter treatment often hinges on how a parent experiences the balance between the overall personal costs of non-treatment and those of treatment.

Society's costs of non-treatment

As a society, we are not sufficiently aware that our communities are less safe and the quality of life for all is diminished because we maintain low standards of care for emotionally and behaviorally troubled children and adolescents. Not living up to higher standards than we currently do has costs that show up indirectly. For example, over-burdened (and under-funded) children's mental health services may not be available to help highly stressed parents and children. As that happens:

- the unaddressed emotional problems of a child may lead to more crises and more use of costly emergency services

- parents' mental health disorders increase and absenteeism at work goes up

- child abuse may go up, creating additional costs for social service agency interventions

- older teens may use illicit drugs to "treat" their anxiety, depression, and anger, and society "pays" the price

- unaddressed emotional and behavioral problems spill over into the school setting:

    ○ Costly extra personnel or specialized programs are required to help untreated emotionally troubled children move forward academically or socially, and not be a major disruptive force in the school.

    ○ These higher costs are reflected in a higher school budget and higher property and state taxes.

    ○ A child who might make it at school and at home with sufficient community support/resources may need a costly residential program.

    ○ A behaviorally troubled child with a learning disorder and unaddressed emotional needs may wind up in a juvenile delinquent lockup.

    ○ The cost for residential care and juvenile lockup facilities (borne by the local and state communities through higher taxes) is great: over $100,000 a year per child in residential treatment programs and more in a lockup.

Under-funding of children's mental health services is very shortsighted and extremely costly in the long run.

To illustrate the long-term costs associated with non-treatment, consider this analogy.

Imagine that a public university decides to build a library. But money is tight. Therefore the administration chooses the lowest bid, hoping that the building could be built for the lower amount of money, even though that seems unlikely. The building is built.

Within a few years, bricks start to fall out of the building. It becomes unsafe to walk near the building and faculty and students become afraid. As a result, the university stops providing library services to the community that it was meant to provide. Professors and students use other resources nearby and charge their transportation and other costs to the university.

When all these are tallied, administrators find that the actual cost of the library, including the needed repairs, far exceeds the highest original bid.

The same is true with under-funding of children's mental health services. The cost of child mental health treatment is relatively easy to calculate and seems high. Yet, the cost of not providing services, although harder to calculate, is much higher. From a community perspective, the expression "pay now or pay later" certainly applies. The future does truly reside in our children. They need better care, and better care costs more than poor care.

Our society could do a lot better with providing help to parents who are seeking treatment for a child. There is a vast discrepancy between the kind of mental health services this country *could* afford and provide for its children and what it *does* provide. This gap is perpetuated and increased by the current (2000–2007) political and social atmosphere, in which politicians are blindly intent on cutting taxes and minimizing the costs of running the government. This means cutting back on public services.

On the scale of where the limited pool of public money should be spent, a low value is put upon community mental health services for children: everything from hospitals, clinics, and residential care facilities to the training of mental health professionals. A higher value is put on military services, weaponry, prisons, and the institutions for the "war" on drugs and terrorism. More public money, either through increased taxes or reallocating money from other areas, needs to be spent on mental health services for children.

To help remedy this situation, you can do the following:

- Support a local or state wide advocacy group that lobbies for better mental health services for children.

- Write a letter to your state and federal representatives indicating your support for more money to improve child mental health services, even to the point of raising taxes for it!

* * *

This chapter brings *Help Your Child or Teen Get Back On Track* to a close. The aim of this book has been to provide you with a broad fund of useful information about your child's emotional and behavioral problems. I hope it has fulfilled its goal. Of course, while the content of this book is similar to what you might receive in a meeting with an experienced child psychiatrist or seasoned child clinician, it is no real substitute for the back and forth exchange of a face-to-face consultation.

APPENDIX: SELF-HELP RESOURCES

I have listed below different sources of information and assistance that you may find helpful. These resources may increase or complement any new learning that you gain from contact with a professional. I have divided this listing into two general areas. The first is information obtained individually: through books, magazines, and the Internet. The second is help and information obtained through participation in a topic focused group.

I strongly support self-help resources and believe that being an informed parent makes you the best and most vital resource for help and advocacy for your child. The professional that you and your child see is a very important starting place for information and understanding, but that person should not be your only source. In this era of "bottom line" approach to health care, you can advocate better for the services your child needs when you are a well-informed parent. While most sources of information are legitimate, you, as the "buyer," need to be thoughtful and cautious in assessing what you learn, especially with information obtained over the Internet. Discuss your findings and the questions that arise from what you find with your child's doctor/therapist. The resources below are ones that I have personally used and recommended to parents or have been recommended to me by colleagues who have made use of these resources in their own practices.

General books on parenting

Raising Resilient Children: Fostering Strength, Hope, and Optimism in Your Child. Robert Brooks, Sam Goldstein (2002). New York, NY: McGraw-Hill.

SOS: Help for Parents. Lynn Clark (1985). Bowling Green, KY: Parents Press.

Parenting Teens with Love and Logic: Preparing Adolescence for Responsible Adulthood. Foster Cline, Jim Fay (1993). Colorado Springs, CO: Pinon Press.

Parenting Your Premature Baby and Child: The Emotional Journey. Deborah L. Davis *et al.* (2004). Golden, CO: Fulcrum Publishing.

Children: The Challenge. Rudolf Dreikurs *et al.* (1974). New York, NY: Hawthorn Books.

Discipline Without Tears. Rudolf Dreikurs *et al.* (1980). New York, NY: Hawthorn Books.

Parenting from the Inside Out. Daniel Siegel, MD, Mary Hartnell (2004). New York, NY: Jeremy Tarcher/Penguin, Penguin Group.

The Hurried Child: Growing up Too Fast, Too Soon. David Elkind (1989). Boston, MA: Addison Wesley Publishers.

The Mother–daughter Project: How Mothers and Daughters Can Bond Together, Beat the Odds, and Thrive through Adolescence. S. Ellen Hawkins and Renée Shultz (2007). New York, NY: Hudson Street Press.

Ties That Stress: The New Family Imbalance. David Elkind (1998). Cambridge, MA: Harvard University Press.

How to Talk So Kids Will Listen and Listen So Kids Will Talk. Adele Faber and Elaine Mazlish (1980). New York, NY: Avon Books.

Siblings without Rivalry: How to Help Your Children Live Together So You Can Live Too. Adele Faber and Elaine Mazlish (1998). New York, NY: Avon Books.

1–2–3 Magic: Effective Discipline for Children 2–12. Thomas W. Phelan, PhD (1995). Glen Ellyn, IL: Child Management.

Ages and Stages: a Parents' Guide to Normal Childhood Development. Charles E. Schaefer, Teresa Foy DiGeronimo (2000). New York, NY: John Wiley and Sons.

The Optimistic Child: Proven Program to Safeguard Children from Depression and Build Lifelong Resistance. Martin E. Seligman (1995). New York, NY: Harper Collins.

Get Out of My Life, but First Could You Drive Me and Cheryl to the Mall: A Parents Guide to the New Teenager. Anthony E. Wolf (1993). New York, NY: Noonday Press.

Specific problem/symptom focused books

Asperger's syndrome

Asperger's Syndrome: A Guide for Parents and Professionals. Tony Attwood (1998). London: Jessica Kingsley Publishers.

Freaks, Geeks, and Asperger's Syndrome: A User Guide to Adolescence. Luke Jackson and Tony Attwood (2002). London: Jessica Kingsley Publishers.

Asperger's Syndrome and Difficult Moments: Practical Solutions for Tantrums, Rage, and Meltdowns. Brenda Smith Myles and Jack Southwick (1999). Shawnee Mission, K: Autism Asperger Publishing Company.

Helping a Child with Nonverbal Learning Disorder or Asperger's Syndrome: A Parent's Guide. Kathryn Stewart (2002). Oakland, CA: New Harbinger Publications.

Attentional problems

Taking Charge of ADHD: A Complete, Authoritative Guide for Parents. Russell A. Barkley (2000). New York, NY: Guilford Press.

Driven to Distraction. Ned Hallowell and John Ratey (1995). New York, NY: Touchstone.

Brainstorms: Understanding in Treating the Emotional Storms of Attention Deficit Hyperactivity Disorder from Childhood through Adulthood. H. Joseph Horacek (1998). New York, NY: Jason Aronson.

Your Active Child: How to Boost Physical, Emotional, and Cognitive Development through Each Appropriate Activity. Rae Pica (2003). New York, NY: McGraw-Hill Companies.

How to Reach and Teach ADD/ADHD Children: Practical Techniques, Strategies, and Interventions for Helping Children with Attention Problems and Hyperactivity. Sandra Reif (1993). San Francisco, CA: Jossey-Bass, a Wiley imprint.

ADHD Book of Lists: A Practical Guide for Helping Children and Teens with Attention Deficit Disorder. Sandra F. Reif (2003). San Francisco, CA: Jossey-Bass, a Wiley imprint.

Anxiety

Helping Your Anxious Child: a Step-by-Step Guide for Parents. Ronald Rapee *et al.* (2000) Oakland, CA: New Harbinger Publications.

The Anxiety Cure for Kids: A Guide for Parents. Elizabeth DuPont Spencer *et al.* (2003). Hoboken, NJ: John Wiley and Son.

Behavior-related problems

The Explosive Child: A New Approach for Understanding and Parenting Easily Frustrated, "Chronically Inflexible" Children. Ross Greene (1998). New York, NY: Harper Collins.

Bullying at School: What We Know and What We Can Do (Understanding Children's Worlds). Dan Olweus (1993). Cambridge, MA: Blackwell Publishing Ltd.

The Defiant Child: a Parents' Guide to Oppositional Defiant Disorder. Douglas Riley (1997). Dallas, TX: Taylor Trade Publishing.

Compulsions and obsessions

Freeing Your Child from Obsessive–compulsive Disorder: A Powerful Practical Program for Parents of Children and Adolescents. Tamar E. Chansky (2000). New York, NY: Three Rivers Press.

The Boy Who Couldn't Stop Washing: The Experience and Treatment of Obsessive Compulsive Disorder. Judith L. Rapoport (1991). Toronto, Ontario: Signet/Penguin Books Canada.

Obsessive–compulsive Disorder (Patient-Centered Guides). Mitzi Waltz (2000). Sebastopol, CA: O'Reilly and Associates.

Eating disorder

When Your Child Has an Eating Disorder: A Step by Step Workbook for Parents and Other Caregivers. Abigail H. Natenshon (1999). San Francisco, CA: Jossey-Bass, a Wiley imprint.

Mood related problems: depression

Growing Up Sad: Childhood Depression and Its Treatment. Leon Cytryn (1998) *et al.* New York, NY: W.W. Norton.

Raising Depression-Free Children: A Parents' Guide to Prevention and Early Intervention. Kathleen Panula Hockey (2003). Minneapolis, MN: Hazelden Information Education.

Helping Children Cope With the Loss of a Love One: A Guide for Grown-ups. William C. Kroen (1996). Minneapolis, MN: Free Spirit Publishing.

Mood related problems: bipolar disorder

Survival Strategies for Parenting Children with Bipolar Disorder: Innovative Parenting and Counseling Techniques for Helping Children with Bipolar Disorder and the Conditions That May Occur with It. George T. Lynn (2000). London: Jessica Kingsley Publishers.

The Bipolar Child: The Definitive and Reassuring Guide to Childhood's Most Misunderstood Disorder. Dmitri Papolos and Janice Papolos (2000). New York, NY: Broadway Books, Random House.

The Ups and Downs of Raising a Bipolar Child. Judith Lederman and Candida Fink (2003). New York, NY: Fireside Simon & Schuster.

Tourette's syndrome

Tourette's Syndrome and Human Behavior. David Comings (1990). Duarte, CA: Hope Press.

Trauma

Children and Trauma: A Guide for Parents and Professionals. Cynthia Monahon (1993). San Francisco, CA: Jossey-Bass, a Wiley imprint.

Miscellaneous—divorce

Making Divorce Easier on Your Child: 50 Effective Ways to Help Children Adjust. Nicholas Long, Rex L. Forehand (2002). New York, NY: McGraw-Hill.

Miscellaneous—meditation

Teaching Meditation to Children. David Fontana and Ingrid Slack (1998). Boston, MA: Element Books.

Other books on children's mental health problems

It's Nobody's Fault: New Hope and Help for Difficult Children and Their Parents. Harold Koplowicz (1996). New York, NY: Random House/Times.

Straight Talk about Your Child's Mental Health. Stephen V. Faraone (2003). New York, NY: Guilford Press.

What It Takes to Pull Me Through: Why Teenagers Get in Trouble and How Four of Them Got Out. David Marcus (2005). New York, NY: Houghton Mifflin.

Psychiatric medication

Straight Talk about Psychiatric Medications for Kids. Timothy E. Wilens (2004). New York, NY: Guilford Press.

The above list of books is a place to start; I suggest you check your local library, bookstore, and friends for other suggestions.

Meditation/relaxation CDs for children and adolescents

"Good Night…Sleep Well" and *"Energy and Me…Relaxation"*
Meditation CDs for children by Dr Roxanne Daleo
www.healingproducts.com/mindworks_kids.htm#relaxation

"Easing Into Sleep" and *"Letting Go of Stress"*
Meditation CDs for older children and adolescents by Dr Emmett Miller
www.drmiller.com/products/body.html#easingintosleep

Magazines

If you have not already discovered magazines aimed at helping with parenting, which have sections addressing common and not so common difficulties and disorders of childhood, here are some suggestions: *Parenting Magazine*, *Parents Magazine*, and *Wondertime*.

Internet

The following are some Internet web sites I've visited and which are quite solid sources of information.

American Academy of Child and Adolescent Psychiatry — This site serves parents by providing information to aid in the understanding and treatment of the developmental, behavioral, and mental disorders which affect an estimated 7 to 12 million children and adolescents at any given time in the United States.

www.aacap.org

American Academy of Pediatrics — Information is provided on raising emotionally healthy children and coping with common behavioral and mental health conditions and stressful life situations.

www.aap.org/healthtopics/behavmenthlth.cfm

Mental Health America (formerly National Mental Health Association) — is an organization to promote mental health and improve conditions for children and adults living with mental health problems. It encourages advocacy, research, and education through its affiliates nation wide.

www.nmha.org

NAMI — (The National Alliance on Mental Illness) is regarded as the nation's largest grassroots mental health organization. Through various activities it offers support, education, and advocacy for people living with mental illness, and their families, as well as raising funds towards research into the causes and treatment of mental illness.

www.nami.org

NOAH: New York Online Access to Health — NOAH provides up to date, unbiased health information in English and Spanish.

www.noah-health.org

About our kids — New York University Child Study Center web site, "About Our Kids," on child mental health offers a variety of resources.

www.aboutourkids.org

Topic focused groups

Online resources can provide an enormous amount of helpful information, and there are chat rooms that provide the opportunity to "talk" with others who are struggling with similar concerns. But, I know that face-to-face group meetings, regularly scheduled and regularly attended, offer a dimension of support and help that is not available through electronic communications. I list some of these groups below and how you might find a local group in which to participate.

Adult children of alcoholics — *ACOA* involves adults who themselves are children of alcoholic families. See *www.adultchildren.org* for more information and consult a local newspaper to find a chapter near you.

Chadd — *CHADD* is a parent led organization focusing on children and adults with ADD/ADHD. See *www.chadd.org/about_chadd.htm* to find a chapter near you.

OC Foundation — Obsessive Compulsive Disorder support groups are available. See *www.ocfoundation.org* to find a chapter near you.

Parents Anonymous — Parents Anonymous is a nation wide organization with local chapters that is focused on helping parents who are concerned about experiencing abusive parent–child relationships. See www.parentsanonymous.org or a local newspaper to find a chapter near you.

There are many other kinds of support groups available. As I indicate above, I suggest you start your search by looking for specific self-help parent organizations in your local newspaper. Also look at your hospital's and clinic's announcement boards, as well as other parts of your health network. You can also explore on the Internet, starting with Mental Health America, in the help section (www.nmha.org/go/help), or the American Self-Help Group Clearinghouse Self-Help Group Sourcebook Online found at www.mentalhelp.net/selfhelp. Remember to read the disclaimer offered on that page before making use of the Sourcebook database. It is a reminder that the Self-Help Clearinghouse does not evaluate or rate the individual self-help groups which are contained in the database.

I encourage you to discuss your experience with your pediatrician, family practitioner, or child mental health specialist.

You are very welcome to offer your comments and suggestions about the book at www.backontrack.kentalan.com.

INDEX